Running Injuries

Jeff Galloway

With David Hannaford DPM

RUNNING INJURY FREE

Prevent and Treat the Most Common Running Injuries

SECOND EDITION

Meyer & Meyer Sport

British Library Cataloguing in Publication Data
A catalogue record for this book is available from the British Library

Running Injury Free
Maidenhead: Meyer & Meyer Sport (UK) Ltd., 2025
ISBN: 978-1-78255-275-8

Aachen, Auckland, Beirut, Cairo, Cape Town, Dubai, Hägendorf, Hong Kong, Indianapolis,
Maidenhead, Manila, New Delhi, Singapore, Sydney, Tehran, Vienna

 Member of the World Sport Publishers' Association (WSPA), www.w-s-p-a.org

Printed by King Printing Company, Inc., Lowell, MA
www.kingprinting.com
Printed in the United States of America
ISBN: 978-1-78255-275-8

Email: info@m-m-sports.com
www.thesportspublisher.com

Manufacturer under the GPSR
Meyer & Meyer Fachverlag und Buchhandel GmbH
Von-Coels-Str. 390
52080 Aachen
Germany

CONTENTS

INJURY-FREE FOR OVER 40 YEARS

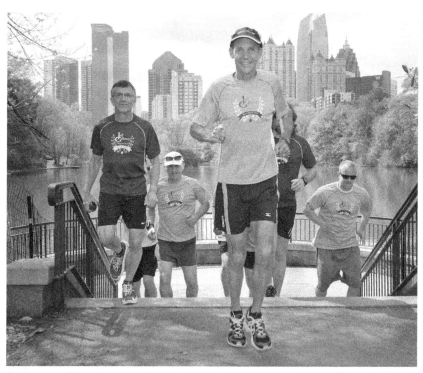

Courtesy of Jeff Galloway.

Over 50 years ago I literally took the first steps in a life-changing experience: I started running. As a fat and lazy 13-year-old, I enrolled in a required conditioning program at my school, fully expecting that running was going to hurt, and that I would quit after 10 weeks of punishment. To my surprise, I felt really good during and after most of my runs. My vitality and positive attitude was better than at any other time of the day. My new running friends were energetic, mentally alert, and fun. As I pushed back the distance barriers, I discovered positive feelings and resources I had never experienced. When I was running correctly, I experienced a sense of freedom and well-being that was wonderful and unique. Running helped me be happy.

I became hooked on running and competition. But male ego and testosterone led me into a series of aches, pains, and significant injuries. Not wanting to give up the wonderful benefits, and lacking perspective, I often went into denial at the onset of an injury and was forced to stop running after a few more runs due to breakdown of muscles and tendons. The worst part was the psychological letdown during every "vacation" from running (about every three to four weeks). The withdrawal from endorphins inspired a desire to eliminate injury. This book is my latest step in that direction.

In 1978 I faced the reality that I would probably never run as fast as I had during my first 20 years of running. My new goal was to stay free from overuse injuries. I'm proud to say that for more than 40 years, I've done this. Chances are, you can be mostly injury free, too. In this book I will tell you the principles and steps that have kept me and over 500,000 clients pretty much away from the doctor's office.

Every week most runners have some aches, pains, injury issues, or questions about whether they have an injury. When I give advice it is from one runner to another. Get medical advice from a doctor who has treated a great number of athletes with the same injury, successfully. In this book, friend, runner, and doctor, David Hannaford, has contributed the info on troubleshooting running injuries and how to treat them. He has a gift for communicating his knowledge in way that those who aren't medical professionals can easily understand.

Both of us want you to understand why injuries occur, how to avoid them and that there are successful ways to prevent and treat them. We want you to gain control over your ailments.

WHY DO WE GET INJURED AND HOW CAN WE AVOID THE RISKS?

In this chapter, I examine why runners get injured and how they can best avoid the risk of injury. In addition, I take a look at how you can stay in shape while injured, how to troubleshoot running form, and how to return to running after an injury, and more.

WHAT CAUSES INJURIES?

Our bodies are programmed to adapt to running and walking by making constant "upgrades" to withstand stress and perform more efficiently. Regular and small increases in workload, followed by recovery periods, promote rebuilding and improved capacity. The factor that is most commonly neglected is rest, but it is crucial. It is during the recovery period that repair and rebuilding occur.

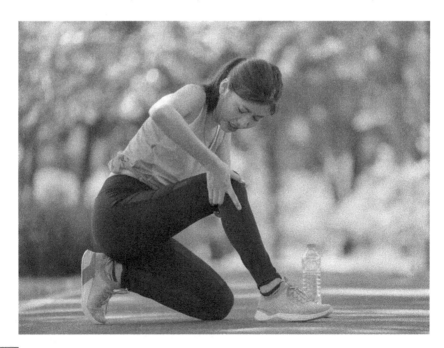

But each of us has a few weak links that take on more stress when we work out. These are the areas that ache, hurt, or don't work correctly when we start a new activity, increase training, or don't provide sufficient rest after a hard workout. In some cases, painkilling hormones, such as endorphins, will mask the damage. Most commonly, exercisers go into denial, ignore the first signs of irritation, and continue training until the stressed area breaks down.

To sustain progress and avoid injury, we simply need to remember that

1. a slight increase in training produces a minor breakdown of tissue;

2. with a sufficient recovery period post workout (usually about 48 hours), the muscles, tendons, and cardiovascular system can adapt and rebuild stronger to handle a higher level of performance; and

3. all body parts continue to adapt in structure, efficiency, and performance when there is an adequate balance between workout stress and rest.

RUNNING IMPROVEMENT CONTINUES IF

- we don't push too far beyond current capabilities;
- we engage in regular workouts; and
- we provide adequate recovery after the stressful sessions.

BE AWARE OF YOUR WEAK LINKS

Most of the aches and pains experienced by my runners and walkers are located in their weak link areas—the muscles, joints, and tendons that take more stress due to our individual range of motion. The process starts during a normal workout when microtears develop in muscles and tendons due to the focused stress of continued movement/irritation of these key parts. The number of these tiny injuries will increase on longer or faster workouts, especially during the last third of a goal-oriented training schedule. But in most cases, the rest period after a workout will allow for healing of most or all of this damage.

COMMON WEAK LINKS

- **Joints**—knee, hip, ankle
- **Muscles**—calf, hamstring, quadriceps
- **Tendons**—Achilles tendon, knee, ankle
- **Fascia**—foot
- **Bones**—foot and leg
- **Nerve tissue**—foot and leg
- **Feet**—just about any area can be overstressed

There is often no sensation of pain during or immediately after the workout because the body has a number of painkilling mechanisms (including endorphins) which will temporarily mask the symptoms. But when a critical mass of these broken fibers has accumulated in one area, you have produced more damage than the body can repair in 48 hours. You are now injured.

WHY DO MICRO-TEARS ACCUMULATE?

- Constant use
- Prior damage
- Speed work
- Too many races
- Doing something different
- Sudden increase of workload
- Inadequate rest between workouts
- Not enough walk breaks during runs
- Stretching (yes, stretching causes a lot of injuries)
- Heavy bodyweight
- Stride is too long

COMMON CAUSES OF INJURIES

It's a physiological fact that the constant use of a muscle, tendon, or joint without a recovery break will result in earlier fatigue and reduced work potential. Continuing to run-walk when the muscle is extremely fatigued increases the quantity of microtears dramatically and is a major cause of injury.

By pacing conservatively and by inserting walk breaks early and often, you will gain a great deal of control over fatigue and injury. You'll empower the muscles to maintain resiliency and capacity. This lowers the chance of breakdown by significantly reducing the accumulating damage that leads to injury. Here are some of the training variables that can be adjusted to avoid injury:

- The pace of the long run is too fast.
- Speedwork segments are too fast for current ability.
- Pace is too fast for the heat.
- Sudden increase in speed, distance, or number of speed repetitions.
- Insufficient rest days per week (three days reduce injury rate most).
- Walk breaks are not taken soon or often enough.
- Stretching causes many injuries and aggravates many more, be careful.
- Changing form or technique.

- Shoes—seldom a cause, but can aggravate a weak link.
- Changing from a worn-out shoe to a new shoe.
- Stride is too long. To improve speed, don't extend your stride, but rather increase cadence by using my cadence drill.
- Trauma—running on a slanted or uneven surface, stepping off a curb, in a hole, etc. This happens rarely, but be careful.

NOTE: Download my Jeff Galloway Run Walk Run App for free, then check out the resources.

AGGRAVATING FACTORS

- **Prior damage**, especially due to accident trauma or perhaps trauma which occurred by playing another sport. It may not be possible for all of the damage to be repaired. In most cases, training adjustments can be made to allow for continued running–walking exercise into the mature years.

- **NOTE:** Studies show that runners have healthier joints and fewer orthopedic complaints than non-runners after decades of running. See my book RUNNING UNTIL YOU'RE 100 for more information.

- **Bodyweight**. Every five pounds of weight gain above average per age puts significantly more stress on the joints and weak links. With much more frequent walk breaks, however, weight stress can be reduced significantly.

- **Speed**. Speed training and frequent racing increases stress on the weak links. Reducing or fine-tuning speed workouts can significantly reduce injury risk. When working with e-coach clients, I have found individual adjustments allowing some form of faster training while managing the risk works in most cases.

- **Stride length**. Longer strides increase risk. A shorter stride may not slow you down if you increase cadence or turnover.

- **Bouncing off the ground**. The higher the bounce, the more stress on the push-off muscles. The higher the bounce, the more shock to be absorbed upon landing. Stay low to the ground, touching lightly.

- **Stretching**. I have not found a single study showing that stretching has benefits for distance runners. Many studies show increased injury risk from stretching. I've also heard from thousands of runners who have been injured or had injuries aggravated by stretching. In general, I do not recommend stretching. There are individuals who benefit from certain stretches, however. Be careful if you choose to stretch, and stick to dynamic movements whenever possible. Stretching is not generally recommended as a warm-up or immediately after running. Trying to stretch out fatigue-induced tightness often results in injury or prolonged recovery.

NOTE: Those who have iliotibial band injury can often get relief from a few specific stretches that act as a quick fix to keep you running. Even when doing these, be careful. The foam roller treatment has been the mode that has reduced healing time for this injury.

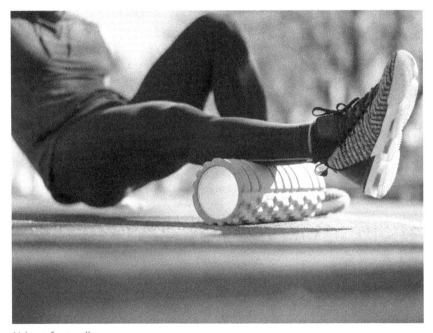

Using a foam roller.

- Continuing to work out when an injury has begun can dramatically increase the damage in a few minutes. It is always better to stop the exercise immediately if there is an indication that you have an injury.

- Avoid certain exercises that aggravate your weak links.

- Prevent foot injuries with the Toe Squincher exercise. Everyone should do this exercise every day to reduce or even eliminate the chance of having a plantar fascia injury or other foot problems. To do this exercise, point your foot down and contract the muscles in the forefoot/midfoot region as you would do with the hand to make a fist. Hold for 6-12 seconds. This strengthens the many little muscles in your feet that provide extra support.

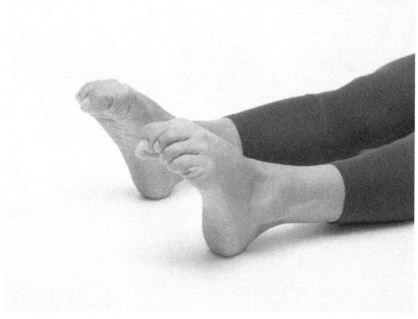

Toe Squincher exercise.

HOW DO YOU KNOW IF YOU ARE INJURED?

Continuing to exercise when you feel that you might have an injury puts you at greater risk for an extended layoff from running. In most of the cases I've monitored, when I suspect that there is an injury, it usually is an injury. Be aware of your weak links. When you notice any of the following symptoms, take at least a day or two off from running.

- Inflammation—swelling, puffiness or thickening.
- Loss of function—the area doesn't work correctly or move normally.
- Pain—if the pain does not go away as you get warmed up and walk slowly, or the pain increases, STOP!

YOU CAN TAKE FIVE DAYS OFF FROM RUNNING WITH NO SIGNIFICANT LOSS IN CONDITIONING

It is always better to err on the conservative side of injury repair. If you take an extra day off at the beginning of an injury, you won't lose any conditioning. But if you continue training with an injury, you may increase the healing time by a week or a month for each day you try to push through pain.

QUICK ACTION CAN REDUCE RECOVERY TIME NEEDED

Some minor irritation may require just one day off from running. As the pain level increases, so does the need for more recovery days, because there is usually more damage.

HOW TO LOWER THE CHANCE OF INJURY

- Insert walk or shuffle breaks from the beginning.
- Work out every other day (lowest rate of injury).
- Avoid faster running or gently ease into faster running.
- Don't stretch (unless you have certain stretches that work for you and don't hurt you).

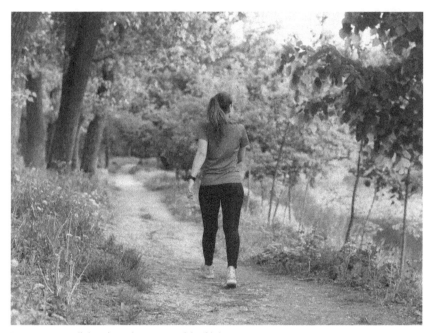

Insert more walk breaks to lower your risk of injury.

STAYING IN SHAPE WHEN INJURED

- Many running injuries will heal while you continue to run if you stay below the threshold of further irritation. Talk to your doctor about this issue to ensure that the healing has started and that you are not irritating the injury as you start back.

- Cross-training—pick an activity that does not aggravate the injury. Walking and water-running are the best for maintaining running conditioning. To hold current endurance, schedule a long walk or water-run session that is the same distance of your long run (same number of minutes you would spend running your current long run). Some runners have been able to maintain speed conditioning by doing a speed running workout in the water once a week.

- Swimming and cycling are good for overall fitness, but don't have a lot of direct benefit to runners.

- Activities to avoid: Anything that irritates the injury.

- If you can walk, walk for at least an hour every other day. Walking will maintain most of your running adaptations. You will receive the same endurance from a long walk as a long run of the same distance.

HOW TO RETURN TO RUNNING

- Check with your doctor to ensure that enough healing has occurred to begin running again.

- Stay below the threshold of irritation. You want to see progress, week by week, in pain reduction.

- Stay in touch with your doctor and ask questions if you suspect that you are aggravating the injury.

- Avoid exercising if you are favoring the injured area or limping. Running in an abnormal way can result in a worse injury in another location.

- If you haven't been exercising, start by walking. Build up to a 30-minute walk (as long as there isn't an increase in irritation).

- Insert small segments of running into a walk (run 5-10 seconds, walk the rest of the minute). If there is no aggravation, you could increase the running segment by 5 seconds while decreasing the walking segment by 5 seconds after using each new ratio for at least three workouts.

- Avoid anything that could aggravate the injured area.

- First training increase goal should be toward increasing the duration of the long run (or walk) by 5-10 minutes every other week. Keep the run-walk-run ratio mostly (or entirely) walking for the first month and slowly increase as the irritation is reduced.

INJURIES FROM RUNNING FORM MISTAKES

While the body adapts and adjusts to the running motion, workouts or races that are long or fast (for you) can result in irregularities in our normal form. Since the body has not adapted to these wobbles, weak links can be irritated. Continued use—using an unaccustomed range of motion—can lead to injury. For more information, see my books GALLOWAY'S HALF MARATHON TRAINING and GALLOWAY'S 5K/10K RUNNING. You can also download my Jeff Galloway Run Walk Run app for free.

TYPICAL FORM-RELATED INJURIES AND THEIR CAUSES

- Lower back pain caused by leaning forward, overstriding, taking too few walk breaks.
- Neck pain caused by leaning forward or placing the head either too far forward or too far back.
- Hamstring pain caused by too long of a stride length or stretching.
- Shin pain caused by too long of a stride length, especially on downhills or at end of run.
- Shin pain on inside caused by overpronating the feet.
- Achilles pain caused by stretching, speedwork, or overpronating.
- Calf pain caused by stretching, speedwork, or inadequate number of walk breaks.
- Knee pain caused by taking too few walk breaks or overpronating.

THE SHUFFLE

The most efficient and gentle running form is a shuffle: The feet stay close to the ground, touching lightly with a relatively short stride. When running at the most relaxed range of the shuffling motion, the ankle mechanism does a great deal of the work, and little effort is required from the calf muscle. But when the foot pushes harder and bounces more, and the stride increases, there are often more aches, pains and injuries.

SPEEDWORK INCREASES INJURY RISK

Time goal runners need to run faster in some workouts, and this means some increase in stride length, a greater bounce, and foot pushing are needed. By gradually increasing the intensity of speed training (with sufficient rest intervals and rest days in between) feet and legs can adapt. But there is still a risk of injury. Be aware of your weak links and don't keep running if there is the chance that you may have the beginnings of an injury (see also p. 30).

CORRECT POSTURE CAN REDUCE ACHES AND PAINS

Posture is an individual issue. Most of the runners I have coached find that an upright posture (like a puppet on a string) is best at any running pace. When runners use a forward lean there is a tendency to develop lower back pain and neck pain. A small minority of runners naturally run with a forward lean with no problems. In this case, one should run the way that is most natural.

SUGGESTIONS FOR RUNNING SMOOTHER, REDUCING IRRITATION TO WEAK LINKS

- Feet should be low to the ground, with each foot only touching the ground lightly as you run.

- Try not to bounce more than an inch off the ground.

- Let your feet move in the way that is natural for them. If you tend to land on your heel and roll forward, do so.

- If you have motion control issues, a foot device can provide minor correction to bring you into alignment and avoid irritating a weak link. A supportive shoe is also needed.

- Maintain a gentle stride that allows your leg muscles to stay relaxed. In general, it's better to have a shorter stride, and focus on quicker turnover if you want to speed up.

- Water-running can help in eliminating flips and turns of the feet and legs—which sometimes cause injuries, aches, and pains. With a flotation device, run in the deep end of the pool so that your foot does not touch the bottom. Even one session of 15 minutes once a week can be beneficial.

MUSCLE CRAMPS

At some point, most people who run will experience at least an occasional cramp. These muscle contractions usually occur in the feet or the calf muscles and may come during a run or walk, or they may hit at random afterward. Very commonly, they will occur at night, or when you are sitting around at your desk or watching TV in the afternoon or evening. When severe cramps occur during a run, you will have to stop or significantly slow down. Medications, especially statin drugs, have been connected to cramping during exercise. If this is a possible cause, talk to your doctor—there may be a medication that allows you to run cramp-free. An over-the-counter salt tablet called S-CAPS has been very effective if bloodwork shows you are low in sodium.

Cramps vary in severity. Most are mild but some can grab so hard that they shut down the muscles and hurt when they seize up. Light massage can relax the muscle and allow it to get back to work. Stretching usually increases the damage from the cramp, tearing the muscle fibers, according to my experience.

Most cramps are due to overuse—doing more than in the recent past, or continuing to put yourself at your limit, especially in warm weather. Look at the pace and distance of your runs and workouts in your training journal to see if you have been running too far, or too fast, or both. Remember to adjust pace for heat: 30 seconds a mile slower for each 5 °F of temperature increase above 60 °F—or 20 seconds per kilometer slower for every 2 °C of temperature increase above 14 °C.

Continuous running increases cramping. Taking walk breaks more often can reduce or eliminate them. Numerous runners who used to cramp when they ran continuously stopped cramping with a 30-second walk break after 30-90 seconds of running during a long or fast run. Check the suggested run–walk strategies in this book or my Jeff Galloway Run Walk Run app.

During hot weather, a good electrolyte beverage (consumed during the day 24 hours after a long or hard run) can help to replace the fluids and electrolytes that your body loses in sweating. Accelerade has been the most effective in my experience. Drink about 6-8 oz every hour for two to four hours as needed.

On extremely long hikes, walks, or runs, (especially during hot weather) the continuous sweating can push your sodium levels too low and trigger a fatigue cramp more quickly. If this happens regularly, a buffered salt tablet has helped greatly—a product such as S-CAPS. If you have any blood pressure or other sodium issues, check with your doctor first.

HERE ARE SEVERAL WAYS OF DEALING WITH CRAMPS

1. Take a longer and more gentle warm-up.

2. Shorten your run segment and take walk breaks more often.

3. Slow down your walk, and walk more.

4. Shorten the distance on a hot or humid day for your maintenance runs.

5. Break your run up into two segments (but not long runs or speed workouts).

6. Look at any other exercise that could be causing the cramps.

7. Take a buffered salt tablet during your long workouts (follow the directions on the label).

8. Don't push off as hard or bounce as high off the ground.

9. During speed workouts on hot days, walk more during the rest interval.

EXERCISES THAT CAN PREVENT OR TREAT INJURIES

Toe Squincher for Plantar Fascia and Foot Injuries

This strengthens the many muscles in the foot, promoting a strong push off, reducing foot fatigue, and reducing foot damage. To do this exercise:

1. Point your foot down and contract the muscles of the foot, which will cause the toes to curl in.

2. Keep the contraction until the foot cramps. Do this 15-20 times a day. Can be done with or without shoes.

Arm Running for Back and Shoulder Soreness and Pain

To do this exercise:

1. Hold a dumbbell in each hand at about waist level, and about 10 inches away from the body at first.

2. Very slowly raise the weight to eye level, maintaining upright body posture and keeping the weight about 10 inches away.

3. Then slowly move the weight back to waist level.

Pick a weight that is heavy enough so that you feel you have strengthened the back, shoulder, and neck muscles, but don't have to struggle as you move the weight back to waist level. Start with one repetition which may be enough for most if the slow motion is slow enough. Those who want to increase can build up to three or four reps, maximum, before increasing the weight.

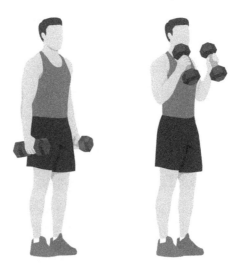

Foam Rolling for the IT Band

This is the only treatment I've found that can speed the healing of the IT band. To do this exercise:

1. Grab a foam roller and lie down on your side, where you feel IT pain.

2. Rest your bodyweight on the roller and then slowly begin moving your body with your hands so that you're rolling from below the pain site to just above it.

3. Roll for 5 minutes before the run, 5 minutes after the run, and 5 minutes before bed at night (probably the most effective).

NOTE: Don't put pressure on the joint. Instead roll on the soft tissue below and above the joint. Apply light pressure over the joint itself.

Ice Massage for Achilles and Other Tendons Next to the Skin

Freeze a paper cup or Styrofoam cup. Peel off the outer layer at the top to form a Popsicle of ice. Rub the ice constantly over the tendon for 15 minutes. The area should be numb after the treatment.

Night Treatments May Help More Than Others

Experts tell me that most healing occurs overnight. If you perform one of these treatments before you go to bed, you may speed up the healing process.

PREVENTING SPEED INJURIES

Running faster than your comfortable pace for that day will increase injury risk. The farther and faster you go in a speed workout or race, the greater the risk. But since you must run faster during some workouts to run faster in races, here are some ways of reducing this risk.

Warm up thoroughly using this warm-up routine:

1. Walk for 3 minutes.

2. Then run and walk for 10 minutes, using walk breaks more often than you would in a normal run. If you use a 90-second run–30-second walk, for example, during the first 10 minutes, use a 1-1 ratio (run 30 seconds–walk 30 seconds or 20–20 or 15–15, etc.).

3. Next, run for 5 minutes starting slowly and gradually picking up the pace to a normal short-run pace. Back off pace and adjust run–walk strategy if you feel irritation of any kind.

4. Finally, do 4 to 8 acceleration gliders. To do these, run for 10-15 steps at a slow jog, then 10-15 steps at a faster jog, gradually accelerate to workout pace over another 10-15 steps and then glide or coast back down to a jog over 30-40 steps. Take a 30-60 second walk–jog and repeat. After 4 to 8 of these, walk for 2 to 3 minutes and start the workout or line up for the race.

- Ease into the speed for the day. Run the first repetition at a pace about 15 seconds/mile slower than you want to run in the middle of the workout. Run the first mile of your race about 15 to 30 seconds slower than your goal pace for that race.

- Insert walk breaks from the beginning. These will vary based on pace and race distance or repetition distance. For more information, see my books, *The Run Walk Run Method®, Third Edition*, (September 2024), *Galloway's 5K/10K Running* (October 2020), and *Galloway's Half Marathon Training* (May 2021).

- The maximum duration of a beneficial walk break is 30 seconds. When walk breaks are longer than this, there tends to be a slowdown during the second half of long runs and races. It is also harder to restart the running after a walk break.

- Walk to recover between speed repetitions. The amount of walking will vary depending upon the distance of the goal race and the pace. It is better to err on the side of walking longer if you feel the need early on, there are more aches than usual, or the temperature is above 70 °F (21°C).

- Never run through pain, swelling, or loss of function—stop the workout. After walking for a few minutes, if the pain goes away, resume the workout with caution. If you start to limp in any way, stop.

- Stay smooth even when tired. If your form is changing due to fatigue, slow down and do check your body alignment. Shortening the run segment can allow you to focus on form on each run.

- Run the last two speed repetition repetitions a bit slower than the pace of the middle repetitions.

- Don't run too many speed workouts, races, or other fast runs too close together. For more information, see the books listed above or my app.

If you are sensitive to your weak links, take the appropriate walk breaks and rest days, and even stop a workout when there could be an injury. By allowing two to five days of rest with treatment, you may avoid serious injuries or a much longer healing layoff.

TREATMENT OF INJURIES

The information in this section has been provided by Dr. David Hannaford.

ABOUT THE LIST OF INJURIES

This list of injuries represents those most commonly seen in my sports injury practice. There are many other less common injuries. The treatments recommended are not a complete list and are changing as time passes. The approach recommended here is from the perspective of a sports podiatrist.

Other practitioners may emphasize different therapies. I have tried to include the treatments that are performed by most other professions, but surely some have unintentionally been omitted. An orthopedic specialist, for example, may have other strategies—especially for knee issues.

It is always best to seek the help of a professional to confirm the diagnosis and rule out complications. This is especially true if the injury does not match the description or if the pain is strong.

THE FOOT AND TOES

TOENAILS—DISCOLORED TOENAILS

TOENAIL TRAUMA

LOCATION OF PAIN

- Pain may be anywhere around the nail plate. In many cases the end of the toe will feel sore.

DESCRIPTIN OF PAIN

- Mild to moderate soreness develops during a run, becoming more sore later. Throbbing may occur at night.

BASIC ANATOMY

- The nails are attached directly to their bed and do not slide over the skin. The skin and nail move forward as a unit.

- Pain occurs when the nail is pushed, pulled, or lifted, separating it from the bed.

- The growth of the nail originates from the cuticle area.

- If the forward part of the nail lifts from its bed, discoloration may occur beneath the nail due to bleeding from the torn vessels into the pocket where the nail no longer attaches. As fluid accumulates, the increased pressure from the pocket becomes painful.

- If the rear part is not damaged (nail origin) the nail can continue growing, pushing out the damaged part over time.

- If the growth area is damaged, the nail will fall off within a few weeks, sitting on the bed until a new nail lifts it loose from beneath.

- Sometimes a very stressful event can produce such a quantity of blood and fluid underneath that a blister forms, bulging out around the border of the nail. The nail may seem to be floating.

- The mildest, yet troublesome, type of nail damage is a chronic thickening, perhaps with yellowing, that never becomes painful, but remains over a long period of time.

CAUSES

- Nails become damaged because of trauma, such as kicking a rock. Runners often produce "black toenails" and other nail damage during long runs during which the toe rubs on the front of a shoe or the insole thousands of times a mile. This can be aggravated by sock fabric bunching or snagging of the nail on the sock. Some runners have a genetic tendency to "claw" with their toes or in the case of a hammertoe, rub against the top of the shoe.

- Athlete's foot fungus can invade a nail and cause thickening and discoloration— usually in multiple nails on both feet. A chronic problem can occur when this fungus moves into a nail damaged by trauma.

PREVENTION AND TREATMENT

- Prevention starts with selection of a shoe that has the right length and shape for the individual foot. If the big toe is squeezed, the nail will catch. If the outer toes are not accommodated, they will rub on the outside of the shoe. Nails grow at different rates, in various degrees of thickness and shapes. Some need a trim every week, others every three weeks. The nails should be trimmed back to the skin junction. Ingrown nails result from trimming too short, so more frequent trimming is the best policy. After trimming each nail, move your finger from the top of the front edge of the nail back. If you feel the leading edge, it will probably catch on the sock or liner or upper as the foot slides slightly in the shoe with each step. Use a good pedicure file to thin or bevel from rear to front on top of the nail so the forward part of the nail becomes very thin. Pedicure files are available at beauty supply counters and at larger pharmacies and are infinitely better than other types of files which result in frustration and wasted time. Some runners tape over the nails during important longer events. Paper tape is best because it is thin and sticks well. Do not place the tape near the rear of the toes because blisters can form where the toe meets the foot.

- When thinning previously damaged nails, use the same approach but work more on the upper surface of the damaged nail. Be careful because these nails may split and become irregular in shape. Take daily care of your nails! One day of neglect with trauma and you'll have to spend a lot more time to repair the damage.

- If nail damage occurs with discoloration beneath the plate, drain it. You may save the nail if you act quickly, reducing pain, and possibly avoiding toenail thickening and warping. If the red, pink, or black discoloration is near the front of the nail, it can be drained with a needle. It sounds painful, but this is not usually the case. Press down on the nail to express the fluid (may sting a little, but icing before and working slowly prevents pain). You can sterilize the needle with a flame briefly, but infection is unlikely with good hygiene afterwards. Line up the needle into the largest portion of the discoloration and push it toward the plate as if you were trying to slide it underneath the nail. You do not need to poke the skin at all. It only needs to enter a very short distance to release the fluid which escapes quickly. This may have to be repeated as the nail bed refills over the first day or so. This usually provides immediate relief of most of the pain. Waiting longer than 48 hours can allow the blood and fluid to become thick and eventually look like a scab as the nail grows out, preventing drainage.

- Discoloration at the back of a toenail that feels "lifted" indicates fluid that can be drained by making a hole in the nail. Heat a safety pin or paper clip to red hot (be sure to insulate your fingers) and penetrate by touching the nail with slight pressure. It will not hurt unless extra pressure is applied. Press only hard enough to slightly penetrate where the discoloration is most dark (the fluid pools there providing a margin of separation). Commonly the fluid is under pressure and will squirt out, providing immediate pain relief. This may also need to be repeated by reheating the pin.

- Protect the nails from infection with antibiotic cream (inserting underneath the nail through the hole if possible), and taping over the hole for a couple of days.

- Fungal nails are more yellow with streaks of discoloration that run from the leading edge to the growth area. There are strong medications that can eliminate the fungus among healthy people. A doctor will need to monitor this, and failures are common. Draining the nail will tend to prevent the spread of the fungus which tends to move into a damaged toenail.

- Many cases of fungal nails heal when the repeated trauma ceases. Treatment can be safely supplemented with topical nonprescription antifungal solutions.

- Medical sampling of the nail is the only way to determine if the fungus is present.

- It may take a year for a big toenail to grow through its cycle. Smaller nails recycle more quickly.

PEARLS

- Severely traumatized nails or nails repeatedly damaged may remain deformed permanently. They can be removed through an office surgical procedure, if necessary.

- Some who have their big toenails removed feel sensitive at the end of the toe on top. Most are quite relieved to have the thick nail eliminated.

- Women with pedicures and artistic nail polish tend to delay trimming their nails and increase the chance of nail damage.

- When a new nail grows in, it can hide beneath a damaged nail for weeks before the damaged nail becomes loose and begins separating. The leading edge of the new nail looks like a hump, but behind the hump is a normal nail. The sharper leading edge does not have to slide over the old nail bed skin. Both grow out together at the same speed.

- A doctor (podiatrist especially) can treat the nail and usually speed the recovery. Podiatrists can also help to maintain damaged nails while the trauma is eliminated, breaking the damage cycle. Ongoing personal maintenance is necessary to prevent damage from regular workouts. A pedicure may help, but usually does not produce the level of thinness needed.

WHEN TO STOP TRAINING

- Usually only a couple of days are needed to recover from nail damage–unless medical treatment was required.

CONSEQUENCES OF RUNNING OR WALKING THROUGH PAIN

- Further damage may occur and other injuries are possible due to compensating and running abnormally.

ANYWHERE ON FOOT

BLISTERS AND CALLUSES

LOCATION OF PAIN

- Calluses are common on the heels, inside of the big toes toward the tip, and at the metatarsal joint. Less commonly they appear at the tip of the second toe and under the ball of the foot behind the big toe, or the third and fourth metatarsal head. The riskiest common spot for a callus is beneath the second metatarsal head, where the toe meets the foot, because this joint is easily injured by too much pressure.

- Calluses can occur anywhere there is mild to moderate friction over a long period of time. They can become painful when they are thick and blisters can form underneath with increased activity.

- Blisters can occur just about anywhere on the foot. They can be painful, but during a workout or race the pain will often decrease, returning afterward.

DESCRIPTION OF PAIN

- Blisters are variable. Sometimes a large blister will have very little pain and other times a small one will be bothersome. Blood blisters (the red, blood-filled type) are usually much more painful because they are deeper.

- Callus pain is similar to that of a bruise. The callus is a foreign object forming on the outside, irritating the skin underneath.

BASIC ANATOMY

- Calluses form when the outer layer of skin (the epidermis) is irritated in a mild way, usually by friction. This increases blood flow and nutrition to the skin cells. They begin to reproduce more quickly and the dead cells (callus tissue) accumulate quicker than they can be worn away. As long as the inflammatory irritation continues, blood flow is present to continue the process. If the irritation stops, the callus gradually dissolves.

- Blisters are caused when the trauma of the friction is so great that a layer of epidermis (skin) separates and fluid seeps into the layer. Blood blisters form when some of the tiny veins that project up into the epidermis are also traumatized. They can break and blood leaks into the separated layer.

- Friction trauma deeper than this should be treated by a doctor. Ulcerations are deeper injuries and very rare in running and walking activities.

CAUSES

- Beginning runners or walkers will almost always acquire a few small watery blisters as mileage increases. With more exercise, the skin adapts by becoming tougher, particularly in the specific areas of the foot that take more pressure and wear.

- There is a wide genetic variability in callus production. A tiny woman may produce larger calluses than an NFL football player. But even those with a strong tendency will experience callus shrinkage if the friction is reduced.

- Recurrent blisters, blood blisters, or large calluses are a sign that the foot is going through stressful and excessive motion. Shoes that don't fit correctly can also be a cause.

- Anyone may get a blister in long or difficult events. Heat, friction, and moisture are the components that cause blisters. Long duration of exposure to these factors or high quantities of any one of them can produce one or more during one workout.

- A rim of hard callus around the heel is nearly always caused by wearing sandals, flip-flops, loose-fitting flats, or an orthotic rim that does not match the heel shape.

TREATMENT

- Calluses and recurrent blisters can be reduced or prevented first by proper shoe fit. Excess pronation can be a cause, for example, if the inner side of the foot is the site. Shoe size and heel counter shape is often related to heel calluses and blisters.

- Callus or blisters beneath the second metatarsal head can be a risk factor for metatarsal phalangeal synovitis mentioned in this book. The same treatment recommended for this condition is also a good prevention strategy.

- A large callus is an irritant itself and should be sanded and softened with lotions (lactic acid or uric acid base are best for thick calluses). This will reduce the motion-caused irritation. Thick calluses can develop a blister beneath them that is very painful and more difficult to treat. Never remove too much of the callus because the underlying skin is tender. A small layer of callus is protective and not irritating. Continue investigating to determine the cause and eliminate it.

- Blisters are treated by draining them as soon as possible – as long as they are not blood blisters. Leave the roof (skin covering) as long as possible for protection to the underlying skin. Make a fairly large opening near the edge and drain the fluid. If the opening is too small it will have to be reopened later. Small scissors, fingernail clippers, and large diameter needles or pins will work. It helps to ice the blister before draining to reduce the pain, although most draining operations are not painful. Sometimes there is a little sting when the roof touches the bed as the fluid leaves. It helps to squirt some Neosporin or similar antibiotic cream underneath the blister for quicker healing and infection prevention. Usually a large band aid can be applied over the area.

- Blood blisters or very large blisters need to be protected for a couple of days. Donuts made of moleskin, or commercial blister products, work very well for this. Eventually a blood blister will open or can be drained after a few days. The infection risk is gone after about 48 hours in most small to medium blood blisters. The blood vessels will seal and repair enough to prevent a pathway for bacteria to enter the blood. There is some risk of further damage, so protection is recommended.

- Once a blister has been drained it is good to cover it for protection when working out to prevent more damage. Simple athletic tape or duct tape can work as long as it is carefully removed, to avoid tearing the roof. Soaking the foot for a few minutes can loosen the roof, and allow you to apply some antibiotic cream. Be sure to place a much larger piece of tape than the size of the blister.

- To reduce the likelihood of unpredictable blisters, use a properly fitting sock of a technical fiber (not cotton). Apply lubrication, such as Vaseline and Body Glide, over the area of blister risk. Silicon-based creams last longer. Applying foot powder to the feet, shoes, and socks can also reduce friction.

PEARLS

- Sometimes in races or very long workouts, a blister will occur for no apparent reason and never happen again.

- Running for long periods with wet shoes is a common cause. If possible, stop and change socks if you sense a problem.

- Extreme dehydration is a cause.

WHEN TO STOP TRAINING

- Blood blisters will often force one to rest and heal, but antibiotic cream can speed the healing.

- Don't run if the pain from the blister or callus forces you to run differently.

CONSEQUENCES OF RUNNING OR WALKING THROUGH PAIN

- Blisters can increase and hurt more if you continue running. But if one is felt during an important race and you have time afterward to recover, you can continue, accepting the consequences. Pain is commonly experienced during a rest break, the warm-up, or afterwards, and hurts less while moving. It is impossible to tell the extent of damage by feel without looking at the blister. Many times they feel like a huge open wound and turn out to be small. Other times very large ones are discovered with hardly any awareness of pain.

TOE NUMBNESS, PAIN, AND TISSUE DAMAGE

RAYNAUD'S SYNDROME

LOCATION OF PAIN

- Usually in the toes, but in some cases the skin on the first or fifth metatarsal-phalangeal joints are involved, especially when there are bunions.

- Athletes are confused because this feels and looks like normal friction damage, but there seems to be no remedy for the pain and irritated skin.

- It is much more common in women than in men.

DESCRIPTION OF PAIN

- The pain can be intense, but it varies day to day. There can be pain without signs of the skin damage.

BASIC ANATOMY

- The vessels in the skin are in spasm and do not provide normal circulation. This prevents the normal healing from friction, so the tissue breaks down gradually.

- This condition can also occur in the fingers, ears, and nose, but the friction is not as great in these areas.

CAUSES

- This condition is genetic, resulting in a tendency to spasm with a shutdown of the tiny vessels that control the circulation to the periphery. This is the body organism's way of preserving heat by shunting the surface blood to the core. Raynaud's syndrome is present when these vessels overreact and then will not release when the stimulus is gone.

- It is not known exactly what makes people develop this problem. It is commonly first noticed in the 20s or early 30s. In some cases it can be related to other diseases such as arthritis, but this is less common.

- Often, only one or two toes will be involved at a time. It occurs in fingers, also.

- Raynauds can occur in cold or warm temperatures, but is most commonly felt during the fall and winter, disappearing when the temperature warms up in the springtime.

- It is speculated that stress is involved, but this is not as common in athletic versions.

- Certain medications can aggravate the disease and stimulants such as caffeine and smoking can trigger it.

- Some versions are so severe that the skin tissue will completely break down, producing open wounds.

TREATMENT

- See a doctor for a diagnosis. Since there is no test for Raynaud's, a doctor will ask questions. There are tests to determine if there are other causes for Raynaud's.

- Initial treatment for mild cases involves keeping the body warm and the extremities protected. In extreme cases, individuals will find relief by spending winters in warm climates.

- Dietary guidelines include no coffee, chocolate, or tea.

- Niacin (Vitamin B3) has produced initial benefit, but loses effectiveness over time. Too much niacin can be harmful. Before supplementing, check with your doctor.

- Doctors may prescribe medications that dilate the peripheral vessels. These can be taken for a few weeks at a time, and are generally safe. Thousands of people take them for years with no side effects for high blood pressure.

- Remember that exercise dilates the vessels and usually helps those with Raynaud's. Runners should protect the toes and forefoot with larger shoes, padded soft socks and lubrication of the foot during workouts.

- For mild cases, try this treatment (get clearance from your doctor before using this treatment if your condition is serious). Fill a pan with water, about 105 to 110 °F. Be careful that it is not too hot (this is about hot tub temperature). Have a pan alongside with ice water. Place the foot in the warm pan for 2 minutes, then the cold for 1 minute. Repeat this 10 times. Be sure to rewarm the warm pan occasionally with a teapot. You are training the vessels in the muscles to open and close by repeating this process. This may need to be repeated on two or three consecutive days. It can be used a couple of times a season if necessary.

PEARLS

- If unusual damage occurs to the toes or forefoot area, consider this diagnosis.

- If you are female in your 20s to 30s and it has never happened before, it could be early stage—see a doctor.

- If you have a tendency to get cold hands and feet and if one or two fingers turn white when others look pink (normal), it is a characteristic.

- It is possible to have pain and blood vessel spasm from Raynaud's without signs of skin damage.

- Smoking is the strongest trigger.

WHEN TO STOP TRAINING

- People rarely have to stop training for Raynaud's, but some need to switch to an indoor area with a treadmill or track if the symptoms are strong.

CONSEQUENCES OF RUNNING OR WALKING THROUGH PAIN

- Common sense rules apply since the only real risk is progressively deeper damage and also decreased sensation over time.

FRONT OF FOOT—BASE OF TOES, OCCASIONALLY TOP OF FOOT

NEUROMA

LOCATION OF PAIN

- Usually in the front of the foot, including the weight-bearing surface at the base of the toes and possibly radiating into the toes, usually the fourth, third, or second toe.

- Sometimes there will be pain on the top of the foot in the same area. In most cases, however, this is felt deep inside or on the bottom.

- In many cases only one of the toes will hurt in shoes, but doesn't hurt when squeezed.

- The pain is usually worse when wearing shoes and relieved by removing the shoe and massaging the foot.

- More advanced cases hurt while running or walking and when wearing everyday shoes.

- If the pain is on top of the foot around an inch behind the toe joint and on the bone, it could be a stress fracture or other bone injury. See a doctor.

- If the pain is at the base of the second toe, even if the toe itself is sore, it is probably not a neuroma.

- If the pain is diffused across the ball of the foot and decreases gradually over hours to days, hurts in other shoes, especially barefoot on hard surfaces, it is probably metatarsalgia and not a neuroma.

DESCRIPTION OF PAIN

- Usually an ache or piercing pain, but may initially be mild. Sometimes cramping of the forefoot or toes may be a symptom.

- Decreased sensation or a numb toe can occur at any time during the injury and sometimes prior to any pain.

- Many people feel a click with or without associated pain at the ball of the foot when walking or running.

- Pain may be intermittent and unpredictable in the beginning.

BASIC ANATOMY

- The injury is caused by irritation or damage to a nerve that travels between the metatarsals and divides at the base of the toes to enter each toe.

- The word neuroma just means enlarged nerve. It is not a tumor since it is composed of the same tissue as a normal nerve. It is produced by physical irritation of the tissue.

- The most common location is between the third and fourth toes. This specific injury is called "Morton's Neuroma" after the doctor who originally described it.

- Neuromas in the inner space between the second and third toes are less common.

- If you suspect a neuroma in any other location it is probably another injury.

- There are neuritises that are nerve irritations in several other locations, but true neuromas are rare elsewhere.

- The actual neuroma injury starts as a mild irritation of the nerve that is similar in size and color to a small toothpick. Continued irritation causes a thickening of the nerve to many times its normal diameter. When the neuroma becomes as large as a pencil, it becomes a candidate for surgery. Less commonly the nerve is irritated to such an extent that it is "strangulated" and becomes smaller than normal and flattened by the pressure.

- Normally, the foot has adequate space between each metatarsal so that the nerve can function without irritation. Over time, the foot may gradually shrink the space between the toes. In some cases this is aggravated by shoes that are too small, over several months or years. One result is the hammertoe shape in which the toes curve upward. In this case, the toe knuckles become rounded and the end of the toe or nail touches the ground rather than the fleshy pad on the bottom of the toe tip. Even mild cases of hammertoe force the ball of the foot to change its weight bearing pattern. In this case the 2nd, 3rd, and 4th metatarsal heads are lower and roll toward one other stretching the nerve upward into the toes—instead of entering straight and flat. This condition is also known as a loss of the anterior arch. When looking straight at a foot from the toes back, at eye level, the plane of the bottom surface of the ball of the foot should be flat. If it is curved, with the center lower, neuromas and foot pain can result.

CAUSES

- Wearing shoes that are too small.

- Wearing elevated heels, especially those with pointed toes.

- Ski boots, bike shoes, and soccer cleats should be considered as frequent offenders.

- Anatomical variations in individuals make them susceptible.

TREATMENT

- Wearing larger shoes for running/walking and every day.

- Sometimes removing the shoelaces and relacing with the lower pair of eyelets left empty can give the extra width needed.

- Sometimes ice massage helps, but there is a low success rate with nerve injuries.

- If it continues to hurt, add metatarsal lifts to your shoe liners. These are oval-shaped pads that are placed at the front of the arch, just behind the ball of the foot in line with the middle toes. Adhesive versions are available at good shoe repair shops if your local running store does not carry them.

- If the problem persists, a podiatrist should construct an insert or place additions on your present footbeds during your first visit. If this approach is partially helpful but not complete, or if long-term maintenance is needed, a true medical orthotic is advised.

- A cortisone injection can be very helpful if a conservative treatment doesn't work. There is always a risk that the cortisone can weaken and shrink connective tissue. But sometimes it's beneficial to shrink the connective tissue that surrounds the nerve and produces the thickening. It is risky to have more than about three injections, and mild cortisone should be used to reduce the risk of shrinking the protective fat pad under the ball of the foot. If injection is used, it should be coordinated with shoe and insert changes.

- Severe cases may require surgery in which a section of the nerve is removed. This is often effective but is usually followed by decreased sensation in a section at the toe junction. Long-term complications are rare if the diagnosis is accurate and good surgical technique is used.

- MRI, X-ray, and ultrasound diagnosis is only slightly useful. False positives and negatives are common.

- Treatments such as acupuncture, foot manipulation, sclerosing injections, and traditional physical therapy may help and are worth considering, but the percentage of success is lower. These are usually recommended if surgery appears to be the only alternative.

- Often it is a "teamwork" of several treatments at the same time that starts the healing process when one singular approach has failed.

PEARLS

- The goal of treatment is to eliminate pain.

- A permanent change of shoe styles and wearing special orthotics can help in reducing pressure on the foot. When this happens, the nerve will probably shrink and remodel itself to its original condition. This process takes many months but can result in fewer shoe restrictions and sometimes the cessation of orthotics.

- Some people, especially those who have had problems in non-sport shoes, or those who had pain for several months to years, may always be sensitive to return of any pain.

- When proper orthotics are used, the pain should improve very quickly. Some feeling of relief is immediate, but over a period of a couple of days further progress is possible. If they are fabricated improperly, the symptoms can even get worse.

- If an injection is required and is performed correctly, there should be a few hours of very strong relief as the local anesthetic that is mixed with the cortisone kills the pain. This can be helpful for confirming the diagnosis. If very little relief occurs, it may mean that another condition is causing the pain.

- It commonly takes several days for an injection to work. Do not assume failure for at least two weeks. The foot may be more sore for a couple of days.

WHEN TO STOP TRAINING

- Pain is an indication of further damage and continued growth of the neuroma. One or two runs with moderate soreness is OK, but no one should continue to train hoping the pain will go away on its own.

- Often the pain is so strong it is impossible to run or walk, or when running causes a harmful compensation. In this case the foot stays tense or rotates through an unnatural range of motion leading to secondary injuries in the knees, hips, ankles, etc.

CONSEQUENCES OF RUNNING OR WALKING THROUGH PAIN

- Ignoring the pain as you continue to run will increase the damage, often producing constant pain requiring surgery.

BOTTOM OF THE FRONT OF FOOT—MAY INCLUDE TOES

METATARSALGIA

LOCATION OF PAIN

- Across the bottom of the front of the foot, or deep inside.

- Does not include the toes. Nor does it include the forward arch.

DESCRIPTION OF PAIN

- Dull ache that can progress to a strong spreading ache.

- Burning is sometimes described, but not tingling.

- Pain may be minor at first and increase as the run/walk continues. The foot will usually remain sensitive after the workout and may be stiff in the morning.

- Incidents that are mild or are in a healing phase may disappear after warming up, and then return during the run at a predictable time or distance threshold.

- Symptoms decrease when taking days off from running/walking.

BASIC ANATOMY

- This is an injury to the second through fifth metatarsal phalangeal joints and related area. Injury may be felt in one or more of these joints. But if at least two are involved the condition is metatarsalgia not synovitis.

- There may be general inflammation, not specific to certain joints.

- This injury is less likely to result in permanent damage or need invasive treatment, but recurrent episodes can foreshadow worse injuries.

- This is commonly experienced by beginners and those who are increasing mileage. The pain will often decrease as the tissue and joints become stronger, and more adapted to running.

CAUSES

- Increasing mileage or intensity too quickly.

- Changing to a shoe that increases supination (from a more neutral shoe), even if the new shoe matches up with the foot type.

- Wearing shoes that are too small or fit too tight.

- Inadequate forefoot cushioning.

- Changing running form to midfoot or forefoot if this is not natural for the individual.

FEET THAT ARE MORE PRONE TO METATARSALGIA

- The same hammertoe (loss of anterior arch) type of foot mentioned in the neuroma section.

- High arched, rigid feet.

TREATMENT

- Go to a technical running store and get expert advice on the right shoe for your feet. Note: make sure that the new shoes have been worn enough to be "broken in." The shoes should also be large enough and long enough for the larger foot.

- Widen the forefoot of the shoe by removing the laces and relacing so that the lower pair of eyelets is not used.

- Purchase a full-length padded insert.

- Icing is helpful after workouts.

- Massage may help.

- Take two to three days off from running to get the healing started.

- Decreasing mileage to half of normal levels for two weeks. Weekly total can increase to normal levels as the symptoms decrease.

- More frequent walk breaks: if one was running 3 minutes/walking 1 minute, drop down to running 1 minute/walking 1 minute.

- Toe squinching exercises.

- Medical treatment is focused on using the right insert for the individual, modified to decrease pressure on the area. By using the full support of the arch, the weight is removed from the forefoot. This approach should be considered if the problem lasts longer than two weeks without any improvement. Unless there is a significant flaw in the foot that is explained clearly, the insert can be a temporary type since this is usually a temporary injury.

- If the problem persists for an extended period of time (6 to 8 weeks) in a new athlete or is a recurrent problem for an experienced athlete, a custom medical orthotic should be considered. Using a well-fabricated device is almost always effective. Seek a second opinion if the orthotics don't relieve the problem after a couple of orthotic modifications.

PEARLS

- Runners/walkers can usually continue training with this injury, if they stay below the threshold of further irritation. If the pain is sharp and strong, it is likely that one has another type of injury.
- If there are symptoms on both feet, diagnosis is probably correct.
- Sometimes the problem is improved by lubricating with Vaseline, body glide, lubricating foot powders, and in extreme situations Hydropel.
- High-quality running socks can help.
- A very high percentage of beginners have this problem and can adapt (with adequate rest between workouts) with no treatment needed.

WHEN TO STOP TRAINING

- It is rarely necessary to stop training for this problem, unless one cannot maintain a normal stride.
- Adding a rest day after symptoms can speed healing.

CONSEQUENCES OF RUNNING OR WALKING THROUGH PAIN

- If the pain persists for more than a few weeks and is ignored, there is probably a structural foot problem or one is suffering from another injury. It is possible for metatarsalgia to develop into a more aggravated condition such as a neuroma or synovitis due to continued stressful training.

THE SECOND OR THIRD TOE JOINT

METATARSAL PHALANGEAL SYNOVITIS

- Also known as capsulitis, pre-dislocation syndrome, plantar plate injury, or metatarsalgia of the front of the foot at the second or third toe joint.

LOCATION

- Inside of the second (or much less commonly third) metatarsal phalangeal joint.

- Pain at the connection of the toe to the foot usually on the bottom or deep inside, but occasionally on top of the joint.

- It is confused with a neuroma, but neuroma pain is between the metatarsals.

- The joint will often swell and feel thicker than the joints on the non-injured foot.

DESCRIPTION OF PAIN

- Achy constant pain that grows in intensity with use, or intensifies if stepping on a rock or bump.

- Pain increases with running/walking, but sometimes will "numb out" during the activity only to return later. Numbing does not mean that the injury is going away. The area is significantly irritated and it is risky to push through this.

- The pain is localized at the base of the joint of the second or third toe, but may extend into the toe and can even produce progressive numb toe.

BASIC ANATOMY

- The initial damage occurs within the joint surrounding the metatarsal head connection to the base of the proximal phalanx of the toe.

- It can start as a simple impact injury from an object on the ground, but it is most commonly a gradual repetitive motion injury because of the improper movement of the toe connection.

- There is a complex apparatus composed of ligaments, tendons, and joint capsule in this area. When any of these tissues are damaged, swelling occurs within the joint producing more damage as the toe bends repeatedly. In many ways this little joint is more complicated than an ankle joint.

- Permanent angulation of the toe toward the big toe is common even after the injury heals because of damage to the joint tissues on the lateral side.

- There is a firm tissue on the bottom of the joint called the "plantar plate" that can become irritated and require an extended healing period, with a tendency to reoccur. In some cases surgery is required.

- There is a variant of this injury in which the joint experiences little inflammation inside, but it is quite sore at the front where it becomes the bottom of the toe. This is sometimes called flexor tendinitis because it involves the long toe tendon that pulls the toe downward.

- In advanced cases the supporting structures become so damaged that the toe dislocates and pops up above the metatarsal. Surgery is then required.

- The swelling that causes the joint to feel enlarged (like standing on a marble) is from synovial fluid which irrigates the joints. The body produces an excess amount when there is inflammation in a joint. The reduction of this fluid is an important part of the healing process.

CAUSES

- Wearing shoes too short or too small. This causes the toe to retract forcing the joint to bend excessively.

- Anatomical progression of hammertoes as mentioned in the section on neuroma.

- A forceful bending of the toe upward, whether suddenly or repetitively as some yoga or work positions require. Forceful downward bending, usually a singular injury, can also cause onset but is more rare.

- Thin soled dress shoes—both men's and women's.

- Too much running/walking before the injury has fully healed. An injury that normally would take a few days to heal can become a long-term problem.

- Excess bodyweight.

TREATMENT

- Initially mild cases may respond to wearing supportive, loose fitting soft shoes at all times. Never walk or run barefooted.

- Get a shoe check at a technical running store. See if the running shoes worn when the problem began were the right model for your feet, were the right size, etc.

- Stop workouts when pain begins. Take several days of rest after a painful workout episode.

- Taking a day or three off at the onset of an injury can prevent having to take weeks or months off later due to trying to push through pain. Be conservative.

- A soft padded insole can sometime allow immediate return to activity in mild cases.

- Use ice massage technique, strategic rest, and avoid bending the toe.

- If the joint feels swollen, put a dab of lipstick on the bottom of the foot at the most tender spot. Carefully slide the foot into a pair of running shoes with loose laces and the factory sock liners inside. Stand up to let the lipstick mark the sock liner. Remove the shoe and pull the sock liner out of the shoe. Cut a circle removing the lipstick mark. This creates a pocket for the sore metatarsal head to drop into, reducing pressure on the joint. This liner can be worn on top of other liners if the shoe is large enough or long enough. It should also be worn in everyday shoes if possible. This "lipstick process" can also be done to a purchased padded orthotic liner as well.

- If the problem worsens over a three- to four-week period, see a doctor.

- X-rays are not very helpful but can monitor a positional change or swelling.

- An MRI can be helpful if surgery is considered.

- Usual initial treatment may involve anti-inflammatory meds to decrease the joint swelling.

- Do not consider an injection unless this is a last resort. Weakening of the joint is likely and delayed dislocation or progressive hammertoe is commonly a result. Injecting the flexor tendon is less risky.

- An experienced doctor can examine the toe noting how much joint swelling is present compared to the other foot, whether the toe slides up and down excessively relative to the metatarsal (drawer sign), whether the tendon at the front of the joint is more painful than the joint itself, or just how easily pain is produced. Analyzing these factors will help focus the treatment strategy.

- Most cases respond to individualized medical orthotic treatment. The orthotics should have a padded forefoot with an additional pocket for the sore area if the area is swollen or protrudes downward. Second metatarsal injuries respond to devices that allow for more supination, if the foot is not already supinated. Metatarsal lifts as mentioned in the neuroma injury section should be used. It is common to require a couple of additional visits to perfect the orthotic even in the hands of an experienced person. The orthotic will probably need to be corrected significantly and regularly for several months. Over time, the amount of correction can be reduced as the injury heals.

- Surgery for this problem is usually not a cure but a salvage operation, allowing some form of activity in a given sport. Surgery is recommended for painful, serious hammertoes or dislocated toes (because the foot would be better than left untreated). Plantar plate repair as a singular procedure has shown inconsistent results in athletes.

PEARLS

- Exercisers are often susceptible to reinjury once they've had this condition, and the other foot should be protected as well.

- This injury is more common in aging exercisers due to a typical falling of the arch that occurs gradually over time. This arch condition is associated with the first metatarsal having upward motion when weight is absorbed which puts more stress on the second joint.

- Many people clutch downward with their toes excessively as a way to hold their arches up if the arches are extra flexible or when experiencing a falling arch. This occasionally occurs during pregnancy.

- A form of immobilization can provide stability to the foot, promoting the healing process: rigid soled hiking boots, padded rigid soled clogs, and sometimes shoes with rocker bottoms or a special shoe modification called a metatarsal bar. These are not made for running/walking exercise, but for daily activities.

- Strengthening the feet while the foot is injured may aggravate the joint. But as soon as healing allows, do some simple exercises such as the toe squinchers. Strong feet are less likely to have this injury.

- If there is little or no progress in healing after extensive treatment, try an even larger shoe than you or the running store would normally consider. This has helped in some slow healing cases.

WHEN TO STOP TRAINING

- Stop training for a few days at the first signs of this injury.

- When you start back, run/walk on grass, dirt, or other softer but stable surfaces.

- Common sense dictates that permanent damage will occur when you abuse a swollen painful toe joint. Stop training if pain cannot be minimized.

CONSEQUENCES OF RUNNING OR WALKING THROUGH THE PAIN

- May end up with a severe hammertoe.

- Gait often changes to avoid pain, causing compensation injuries in other areas. These can be much worse.

- Synovitis may also produce neuroma injuries requiring treatment for two injuries. The swelling and inflammation in the area can damage the nearby nerves.

PAIN IN OUTER TOP OF FOOT AND UP TO ANKLE CREASE

EXTENSOR TENDINITIS

LOCATION OF PAIN

- The most common version is a broad achy feeling across the outer top of the foot and up to the ankle crease. It may radiate almost to the toes.

- The second type of pain is located along the top of the foot extending toward the big toe. It may also appear at the ankle crease. This may be achy and a little sharper.

- If the pain is strong or confined to a small area, it is not this injury.

- The pain is on the surface and not deep in the bones.

DESCRIPTION OF PAIN

- The pain is aggravated by workouts, but decreases with rest.

- The pain may be reduced when the foot is lazy, does not push off, and lands fairly flat.

- Pain at the ankle crease in the front may be localized to a tender spot, sometimes with a bump.

BASIC ANATOMY

- The tendons on the top of the foot pull up on the toes and lift the ankle upward. They prevent the foot from slapping onto the ground when the heel makes contact.

- They function very well when the foot is straight. If the foot is tilted outwardly (supinated) or inwardly (pronated), the load and demand is increased on individual tendons. Usually the force is divided evenly through all of them.

- Tendons become overworked when they are pushed harder than the current level of conditioning, even if the foot is straight. This is usually due to going longer, faster, or running too many fast runs during a short period.

- The pain is caused by irritation of the tendon tissue, inflammation of the sheaths they slide through, and is sometimes due to the shoe pressing on them.

- Shoelaces can damage the tendons at the ankle crease and fibrous tissue can form a bump in this area.

CAUSES

The most common cause is too much supination or pronation. This overloads the outer or inner tendons, they fatigue and then become damaged.

- A mileage increase, particularly too quickly without enough rest between workouts. This is more likely to be the cause if the pain is directly on top or in the direction of the big toe.

- Running hilly terrain more than in the recent past.

- Calf muscles that are unusually tight. This makes it harder to lift the ankle in front. Shortening the stride can reduce the irritation.

- Running with a stride that is too long.

- Running on a soft or irregular surface.

- Wearing high heels is a cause for women, because the key tendons can become overworked. Tight calf muscles are often the result of wearing such shoes.

- Pressure on the tendons due to the lacing of a shoe, or the design of the shoe. The ankle crease is a key pressure area.

- Lacing the shoes too tightly at the ankle or too far up the ankle.

TREATMENTS

- Icing is very helpful—constantly rub an ice chunk directly on the tendon for 15 minutes each night.

- If the soreness is on the outer side of the foot, a more stable shoe is needed. If new shoes were recently purchased, they may allow the foot to supinate more than needed. Many times this is not visible to the person evaluating the stride. Very small differences may be the cause. The outer tendons not only lift and lower the foot, they also lift and tilt the outside of the foot.

- A very slight amount of outer tendon soreness is common with adaptation to new orthotics or a change from poor shoe to a better shoe. This should be very mild and disappear in a couple of days when training is reduced, without having to rest completely.

- Pain in line with the big toe is possible during a mileage increase. A more stable shoe and proper arch support can manage this and may eliminate the pain. The tendons on the inner side of the top of the foot help prevent pronation and keep the arch from flattening too much. They also lift and lower the ankle.

- For pain at the ankle crease, the same pronation and supination suggestions apply. In many cases, simply loosening or changing the lace pattern can help. It is surprising how much protrusion of the tendons occurs as they tighten, even when there is no sensation of pressure on them while lacing the shoes.

- A doctor may prescribe physical therapy treatment for tendinitis, which can be helpful. If there is a bump on the ankle tendons, a doctor may suggest an injection to dissolve it. It's best to avoid this because it can weaken the connective tissue and cause permanent damage. In rare cases the bump is caused by a fluid filled cyst called a ganglion (not fibrous tissue). A knowledgeable doctor can usually identify this by examination. It is safe to drain this if needed, but it often disappears naturally. It is very common for ganglionic cysts to reappear after draining repeatedly. It is best to leave them unless they are irritating and bothersome. Composed of normal tissue, ganglionic cysts result from defects in the tendon sheath or joint capsule, allowing it to balloon outward, attracting the normal fluid found within joints and tendon sheaths. They will sometimes become firm over time and be mistaken for fibrous bumps.

PEARLS

- This type of pain is often diffuse and hard to locate.

- The quantity of pronation or supination needed to cause this soreness is very small and easy to overlook.

- If a bump has occurred on a tendon, it may take months to go away. If there is no pain do not worry unless it grows, turns red, or is very large.

- If the pain becomes centralized to a small area on the forefoot, a stress fracture should be suspected—see a doctor.

- Stop training if the motion of the stride, or moving the foot and ankle up and down while sitting, causes a feeling of sticking or makes a "celery breaking noise." This is known as crepitus and it means the tendons are inflamed so they do not slide normally along their sheaths or tunnels. Even proper foot positioning can cause increased damage. Regular icing and rest is needed, until the inflammation and sound have gone away.

CONSEQUENCES OF RUNNING OR WALKING THROUGH THE PAIN

- A single workout or race is unlikely to cause worrisome damage, but ignoring the pain over a period of time can allow the problem to progress from mild tendon soreness to crepitus and more extensive damage requiring extended rest from training.

- Most people train through this injury as long as common sense running/ walking rules are used and action is taken to correct the cause. Stay below the threshold of irritation.

FOOT—FRONT TO MIDDLE

STRESS FRACTURE OF THE FOOT

LOCATION OF PAIN

- There are several locations of stress fractures in the foot, but there is only one type that athletes can identify themselves. Metatarsal stress fractures are common and can often be self-diagnosed. The pain is located on the shaft of the metatarsal behind the joint. It is usually felt on top, but may be deep inside. The second is more common than the third. The fourth is more rare. I have only seen a couple of first in my entire career, and the fifth is a unique injury that should not be self-treated and hurts in a different location.

- The pain is usually reproduced by pressing on the metatarsal bone from the top. Bend the toe downward and note how the knuckle responds. The pain can be 1/2 inch to about 2 inches behind this joint. If the pain is anywhere else it is not a classic stress fracture.

- After about two weeks a bump can usually be felt on the metatarsal in the location of pain.

DESCRIPTION OF PAIN

- Stress fractures can occur without knowing it. The pain can begin after a workout, during the first part of the next workout, or after sitting and sleeping.

- The pain can also begin during a workout, sometimes in a very short period of time. The pain can become strong. This type of stress fracture is easier to identify because it is obvious, but it also usually means the damage is greater.

- Many times there can be a low-grade ache that does not really hurt much for as long as a week or two, only to become quickly more sore and obvious. This is usually the time that a stress syndrome becomes a true stress fracture.

- The pain is described as an ache, sometimes piercing. The pain can vary from the mildest form that only hurts with exercise, to intense pain that forces one to use crutches for walking.

BASIC ANATOMY

- The injury occurs when the load on the bone exceeds its strength. It can begin as an inflammatory process within the bone or its outer layer. This is nature's way of making the bone stronger by increasing the blood flow, sending repair and remodeling cells into the area. The pain is a reminder for the body to avoid the damaging motion. It is possible to have only mild pain and with luck people often continue to train and the injury does not progress. It may progress and get worse, however. It may require only a couple of weeks to heal from this stage.

- The injury can progress to the point that swelling or bleeding separates the coating of the bone from the bone. This is more painful and many people stop and heal during this stage. It takes almost as long as a true stress fracture to heal this type of damage—usually about five or six weeks.

- The next stage involves damage to the outer layer of the bone. Usually only one side of the bone is involved. This is a true stress fracture, but the mildest form. After about two to three weeks a tiny crack is usually visible on an X-ray. The pain is usually present with daily activity, too painful to run, but not so painful to cause a limp or need crutches for walking. This usually requires six to eight weeks to heal.

- It may progress to a transverse surface crack running all the way from one side to the other. This is more painful and may cause limping during everyday activity. It requires about eight weeks to heal, but rarely as few as six.

- Although it can occur as a typical stress fracture, it is possible for the initial injury to be a true fracture with immediate X-ray visible crack across the bone. Often separation of the pieces or overlap may occur. These are quite painful and require some type of immobilization. Depending on the displacement and the extent of damage, these require from 8 to about 12 weeks to heal.

- Healing does not mean the bone is completely normal. It means that a bridge of bone has connected the separate pieces enough to allow the force of running/walking to be safe.

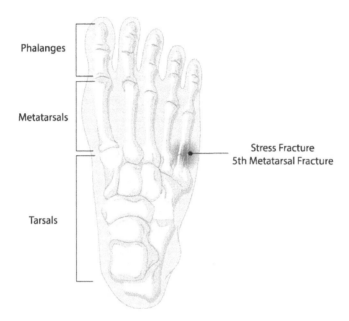

Phalanges

Metatarsals

Stress Fracture
5th Metatarsal Fracture

Tarsals

- The bone can continue to remodel itself for as much as a year. Most doctors feel the bone is actually stronger after a stress fracture heals completely.

- The metatarsal is usually elevated at the joint after stress fractures heal. So the end of the bone lifts slightly as it heals. This is true even for mild stress fractures, but is very evident in the worse types. The consequences can be beneficial if the bone was lower than the others to begin with, but sometimes the force of exercise will be transferred to the adjacent metatarsal and (rarely) a second stress fracture could result.

CAUSES

- Excessive mileage or intensity of workouts prior to the body adapting.

- A singular event that exceeds the current level of the skeletal and muscular fitness of the athlete.

- An overload of the foot because of a change in shoes or surface or running form.

- Poor bone density.

TREATMENT

- Most cases can be treated with rest, supportive shoes, minimizing walking, and icing for the soft tissue portion of the injury.

- If the foot hurts too much to walk with a normal gait, an X-ray is strongly advised to rule out a complete fracture.

- A cast or special boot is not usually needed for mild to moderate stress fractures unless the pain prevents normal activity. Fortunately this pain is also an indicator of the extent of the fracture. More pain means a more severe fracture. A doctor will know how to make the foot more comfortable.

- During the first two to three weeks the pain is at its worst. Consider a stiff soled shoe like a hiking boot, or shoe with lots of padding during this time.

- After about three or four weeks the pain will improve, but do not increase activity yet. It is possible to begin wearing a normal shoe at this time.

- At about six weeks, if the pain is almost gone in normal activity, it is OK to try a test workout. On a flat surface a 20-minute test is possible. Pain means stop. Don't do more than 20 minutes because a delayed reaction is common.

- If there is no pain, a gradual return to training can begin. A feeling in the foot of a "presence" in the injured area is fine and will persist for a couple more weeks. Any form of pain is not acceptable and rest should continue if this is the case.

- Wait one full week and repeat the test. Healing happens quickly and one week is often sufficient to make a difference. Don't be discouraged.

- Doctors often say six to eight weeks of no running, but eight weeks is a minimum. It is common to take up to 11 weeks. If pain persists, see a doctor to rule out complications.

PEARLS

- A single stress fracture is not a reason to suspect bone density problems.

- Reinjury is common because people try to increase training too fast during the recovery.

- Many runners try to run through mild stress fractures, which are sometimes not discovered unless X-rays are taken for other reasons. This is not a good idea, and those who get through this without more damage are lucky.

- Treatment modes that promote healing are pulsed ultrasound, electromagnetic, or electric. These have been studied with inconclusive results in the healing of metatarsal stress fractures. Poorly healing fractures seem to be helped by these.

WHEN TO STOP TRAINING

- Ideally one should rest when this injury is diagnosed.

- If pain emerges after resuming training, taking another week of rest may prevent a complete reinjury to the bone.

CONSEQUENCES OF RUNNING OR WALKING THROUGH THE PAIN

- Progression of the injury is probable. A mild stress fracture can become a complete fracture.

- Many athletes who are training for a significant goal decide to take the risk and run with a mild stress fracture (moderate or severe fractures are too painful). Some make it through, but many aggravate the injury, requiring a lot more rest. Unfortunately, a mild stress fracture can become a serious true fracture within two to three strides.

BEHIND BIG TOE—TOP OF THE FOOT AT THE INSTEP

FIRST METATARSAL-CUNEIFORM AREA

LOCATION OF PAIN

- Pain is focused on the top of the foot at the instep, which is the high point ahead of the ankle in line with the big toe.

- Sometimes the pain radiates up from this point, and toward the big and second toes.

- There may also be deeper pain within the foot, but in the same location.

DESCRIPTION OF PAIN

- Pressing on the area may cause pain.

- Shoes that are laced tightly will cause pain.

- Deeper pain is made worse when wearing poorly supporting shoes or when running barefoot.

- Pain on top can sometimes be intense, burning, and is often mistaken for a stress fracture.

- The deeper pain is achy and increases after activity.

BASIC ANATOMY

- This area is the junction where the first and second metatarsals meet the midfoot bones. Many people have a firm bump on top of the foot in this area. It is often present on one foot and not the other. Many have had it as long as they can remember but most have noticed a gradual growth through the years. Pain may be present without a bump.

- It is possible for the bump to grow very quickly with strong, direct pressure, such as that from a poorly fitting ski boot or among surfers who kneel on the board and rub the top of the foot in this area. A rapidly growing bump appearing in a runner or walker should be evaluated by a doctor and often turns out to be a soft tissue injury.

- Sometimes the bump is pointed and sharp. This is a type of bone spur, indicating greater motion in the joint with further damage and a longer history of irritation. If this is present, try to avoid irritating the area. If shoe pressure can be avoided, removal may not be necessary.

- There are two nerves that rest against the bump on top of the bone: the deep peroneal and the medial dorsal cutaneous nerves. They are easily aggravated by pressure.

- There is normally very little motion in these joints. Too much motion can irritate them.

CAUSES

- By far the most common cause is pressure from above. Shoelaces cross over this spot and press directly on the bump and nerve.

- Everyday (street) shoes often cause this problem–especially slip-on shoes and boots. Many times feet expand during warm-weather exercise, when wearing loose-fitting shoes. When cold weather arrives, the boots are suddenly too tight. Quality loafers and boots will last for years, but the feet change during this time. Many loafers press directly on the bones of the foot.

- High arches with high insteps are especially prone to pressure from above.

- Many people feel they need to tighten their laces because they feel more supported, which is not always the case. Tightening the shoe right before a run can aggravate the pressure on the foot, because feet will swell during a run. The foot slides toward the laces as it contacts the ground with each step. This repetitive pressing against the foot and nerve will trigger the pain. The shoes may not feel tight until after the first mile or so.

- Inserting a new orthotic can be a cause. In this case, the foot device raises the foot and the instep presses on the shoe. This may be only experienced in sports shoes. Shoes should be relaced from the very bottom when new orthotics are used. This may seem like a waste of time, but it prevents injuries.

- Deeper pain is produced when one or more joints become irritated. This happens when the arch collapses or falls. These joints are like a bridge. The bottom of the joints is stretched and the tops are compressed together, and the pressure causes the bone to thicken, producing bumps on top. This is a good thing up to a point because it blocks further sagging of the joint. After a certain buildup, however, the pressure and extra motion damages the surfaces of the bones within the joint and the pain is similar to that of arthritis. This is a sign that a spur may be present.

- When there is deeper pain in the joints and there is a bump on the underside, it is often due to the collapse of the "bridge," with its supporting ligaments. During the gradual fall, the connective tissue pulls on the bones as the joints try to open up. This can stimulate bone growth with arthritic bone spurring on the bottom.

TREATMENT

- The first treatment is to remove pressure from the top of the foot in this area. Wear open shoes or sandals during the day. Relace tie shoes so that the laces don't cross on top of the sore area. Do the following when relacing the shoes:

  1. Put the shoe on and press on the tongue area to locate the sore spot.

  2. Take the shoelaces out and relace, starting at the bottom. When the laces reach the eyelets at the sore area, pass the lace into the eyelet on the same side as previous without crossing over where the sore area is present. Sometimes this needs to be done for two sets of eyelets because the pain is greater or the eyelets are close together.

  3. Relace normally above the sore area. This provides a square patch of the padded tongue of the shoe with no crossing laces over the sore area. If there is doubt about which eyelets are to be blamed, it is the pair just below or directly on top. It is not the pair above the sore spot.

- This elimination of top pressure can help the deeper pain, because the top of the foot is sensitive to any type of pain in this area. If the nerve is irritated, immediate relief may not occur. In this case, continue this lacing pattern for at least a week before trying another lacing plan. Nerves heal very slowly. A sign of progress is often a reduction of pain after the first mile or two.

- Deep pain usually requires support from below using good arch support. Mild cases may heal with better, more supportive shoes and perhaps off-the-shelf orthotics. Elimination of excessive pronation is helpful, but not usually adequate as the only form of treatment.

PAIN THAT IS DEEP INSIDE THE BIG TOE JOINT

BIG TOE PAIN

LOCATION OF PAIN

- The most common injury of the big toe is in the joint where the big toe meets the foot. Most commonly the pain is felt deep inside the joint, but there may be some tenderness on top of the joint and toe.

- If it hurts almost entirely on top, the injury is called hallux limitus.

- If it hurts almost entirely on top and the joint is enlarged on top with limited ability to bend the toe upward, the injury is hallux rigidus.

- If the joint hurts only on the bottom, it is sesamoiditis injury.

- If it hurts on the inner side of the joint toward the other foot and there is an enlarged joint, it is a bunion.

- If it hurts at the joint near the back of the toenail, it is an injured interphalangeal joint and not the same injury syndrome in this section.

- Toenail or end of toe soreness is covered in the nail damage section of this book.

DESCRIPTION OF PAIN

- The pain is usually achy and starts as a dull feeling that grows.

- Running and walking usually causes the pain to increase during the workout as an achy feeling. In most cases, the pain decreases over several days of rest. The pain may be on the surface or on the joint, but it may also be surface pain or located near or on the bunion bump (if present).

- Pain that hurts with everyday activity and does not go away after weeks of rest from running/walking is more serious and should be evaluated by a doctor.

- Less common is an intense throbbing pain that is especially noticed at night and is not directly related to workout, called gout. This is the result of a process where production of a chemical that is normally present in the body increases significantly. The big toe joint is a common target for this substance. The body then attacks the "crystals" of this chemical as if they were irritating foreign objects. This damages the normal tissue and causes pain, redness, and swelling. Any sore big toe can hurt at night and feel stiff upon awakening, but gout pain is intense and increases at night.

- Sesamoiditis is noted by pain on the bottom of the foot at the base of the big toe, beneath the joint, that may feel like bruising—sometimes with sharper pain qualities. Sometimes the area can swell and feel thicker. If this occurs, it is a worse injury, sometimes a fracture. See a doctor.

BASIC ANATOMY

- Pain is caused by abnormal bending or hinging of the big toe upward where it joins the end of the first metatarsal bone. This joint is designed to allow the big toe to hinge straight up and down. Any sideways force is harmful. Some people are born with a rounder shape at the end of the metatarsal which allows the toe to move from side to side very easily. These individuals are more likely to develop a bunion as well as pain in the joint.

- Abnormal movement of the first metatarsal can cause toe joint pain. Doctors diagnose this problem by pushing up on the bottom of the foot beneath the base of the big toe to see if it moves upward more than usual. This hypermobile first metatarsal causes hallux limitus and eventually hallux rigidus. In many cases, the big toe is longer than the second toe, but not always. The rising of the metatarsal tightens the toe joint, preventing the big toe from gliding around the hinge. This forces the top of the toe bone to collide forcefully with the top of the metatarsal bone when the big toe tries to bend upward. Over time, this stimulates the bone to thicken as extra calcium is deposited on top, sometimes forming spurs. Cartilage on the surface, that protects the ends of the bones, can wear down—a form of arthritis. In an advanced stage of hallux rigidus, the big toe loses its ability to hinge, resulting in a perfectly straight big toe.

- Pain on the bottom of the big toe joint is usually the result of an injury to two small bones called sesamoid bones that are positioned side by side, directly beneath the joint, enclosed within tendons that connect to the bottom of the big toe bone. They function as tiny kneecaps except that the force of pushing off, combined with the weight of the person directly on top, can be very stressful. They slide in grooves lined with cartilage. Impact or repetitive force can result in pain. Less common, but often overlooked is the continued and excessive pulling of the tendons that enclose them. This occurs most commonly to the sesamoid bone that is nearest the second toe. The same hypermobile first metatarsal that causes hallux limitus causes this as well.

CAUSES

- Excessive pronation is the primary cause. This is especially true when it occurs after the heel starts to lift—a condition called "propulsion pronation" or "late mid-stance pronation." This often occurs inside the shoe and has no visible signs. The repetitive motion of running and walking, as the distance increases, results in irritation.

- High-arched feet are more likely to put extra pressure on the ball of the foot under the big toe base. This triggers impact-caused sesamoid pain, and is not related to pronation.

- Those with bunions are likely to have pain because the joint no longer works correctly. The size of the bunion is not related to the quantity of pain, however.

- Gout can be triggered by the same motions that produce other types of big toe pain, but high uric acid levels must be present. This "improper motion triggered version" of gout is often overlooked by non-sports doctors. Uric acid is elevated by many factors. Certain foods, alcohol, medications, and an inherited inability to process uric acid are causes. Dehydration, especially over a long period of time can be a trigger. This is common in athletes who fail to rehydrate from their workouts on a regular basis.

- Shoes that are too narrow or too small can be a cause of all of these problems. Those who have longer big toes need to provide sufficient room at the end, even if this results in excess space for the other toes. Some shoes are too pointed in the front, forcing the big toe to be pushed toward the second.

- Shoes with poor forefoot padding can cause sesamoid pain.

- Everyday shoes should be fitted in the same way as sports shoes. See the shoe section in this book.

TREATMENT

- Icing helps.

- Dehydration increases soreness from any of these conditions. Consumption of eight glasses of water or sports drinks per day is recommend. Remember that a cup of coffee or soft drink results in only half a cup of fluid due to the diuretic effect of caffeine.

- All of the big toe injuries, except sesamoid pain in higher arched feet, are helped by reducing pronation. Low- or average-arch-height sesamoiditis is helped by decreasing pronation. Consider more stable shoes and off-the-shelf orthotics.

- Sesamoiditis (especially the high-arched variety) responds to shoe/insole padding and correct shoe fitting (size and shape).

- Pain that began with impact to the big toe, causing joint pain (or underneath), should be seen by a doctor if strong or persistent.

- Any strong pain should be seen by a doctor.

- Sometimes in mild cases a toe spacer between the first and second toes can help the joint to recover. They are difficult to cope with during workouts. But wearing them during everyday activity can speed the healing. They are found in pharmacies.

- Wearing open-toed shoes during the day can be helpful, but avoid unstable, poorly-supporting shoes such as thin sandals or flip-flops.

- Hallux limitus, bunions, and strong sesamoiditis can very effectively be treated with medical orthotics, which can prevent progression over the long term. Pain is a sign of damage and progression of structural damage increases the effect of the injury in every way. This can result in spurring, drift of the big toe, and sesamoiditis can develop into a fracture. Maintaining improved foot positioning with custom medical orthotics is important.

- If the pain cannot be eliminated with shoe changes, off-the-shelf inserts, icing, or rest, see a doctor. Possible treatments involve X-rays, injection, immobilization, medical orthotics, and surgery.

- X-rays can determine if there is joint damage, a fracture, and a change in big toe position.

- An injection of cortisone is acceptable if it is a single injury that has become quite sore. This is especially true for sesamoid injuries, joints already showing signs of spurring, and gout. Multiple injections should be avoided, and this treatment should be coordinated with expert shoe fitting and orthotics.

- Immobilization is best for traumatic injuries such as hitting the toe against a rock, or impact damage to the sesamoid bones. X-rays for sesamoid injuries are often confusing because many people are born with two or three piece bones which may look like fractures. An experienced doctor can tell the difference. If there is a fracture, a cast or removable cast boot will probably be recommended. This will probably fail to heal the fracture. Experience has shown that sesamoid fractures almost never heal unless the person is below the age of 20. Over a long period of time, with rare exceptions, these problems become painless as the pieces separate and the edges smooth. This can require more than a year. During this time it is possible to run or walk, but well-constructed orthotics are needed, along with expert shoe fitting. Periodic soreness is normal. Track athletes, serious racers, and elite athletes tend to keep pushing into greater damage and are much more likely to need surgery. Without surgery the pain should gradually disappear, but a sufficient period "below the threshold of irritation" is needed. In rare exceptions if the pain persists or remains, surgery to remove the sesamoid bone is performed. The bones serve a purpose and changes in foot function may occur after surgery. The big toe may drift and become a bunion or the toe may develop a contracture and look like a hammertoe. This does not always happen but it is common.

- The X-ray may show spurring on top of the joint. If there is a large spur and the joint looks damaged, it is better to try every conservative treatment possible before considering surgery. These joints usually have a decreased range of motion, and surgery cannot return the joint to normal use. Indeed, the ability to run or walk at a high level will probably not be possible after surgery. There is hope that over several years the damaged joints can adapt with a decrease in pain. In advanced stages the big toe cannot hinge at all and adjacent joints can take over most of the work.

- If the joint looks normal but there is spurring, loss of range of motion, and pain, surgery is a much better option. These procedures have a greater chance of success due to the relatively simple act of spur removal. It is commonly believed that the removal of the spur and expert fitting of shoes and orthotics can leave the toe less likely to develop further problems than by ignoring the spur.

- Even when the X-ray reveals a bunion, there is often little or no pain. The toe may be angled very strongly with a large joint prominence. It's common for people with the same size bunion to have a wide variance in levels of pain. Sometimes a small one is much more painful. Experienced doctors know what causes the pain and do their best to eliminate the factors, suggesting surgery in some cases.

- Bunion surgery, often done for cosmetic or shoe limitations, results in permanent damage among a certain percentage of patients. Particularly sad is the situation of a painless toe before surgery and a permanently painful one afterward.

- Surgery is recommended under three conditions: If pain persists, despite proper conservative treatment (including shoe compromises and orthotics) the risk is acceptable. Additionally, if a very rapid progression in bunion size occurred with or without much pain. It is much easier and the results are better when the toe is surgically adjusted before it has adapted to an adverse position. Finally, if the big toe is angling toward the other toes so strongly that they are also beginning to drift sideways or contract. There can be an injury chain reaction with pain that is permanent if left untreated. This surgery is very difficult and requires multiple procedures to correct toes and the bunion. It is best to stop the progression by correcting the bunion first, which often allows the other toes to straighten without surgery.

PEARLS

- For best results, full-length orthotics are used, with correction extending to the toes.

- When the pain has been eliminated for a couple of months, the joint can begin to tolerate many things that previously caused pain. Having had one incidence of this injury usually means a person is vulnerable to reinjury.

- Some doctors will often suggest that bunion surgery will only require six to eight weeks before returning to workouts. This is usually not true, and it can be harmful to return to exercise before the healing has been completed. It is best to be patient and ease back into workouts when the pain is gone.

- Bunions are not only caused by wearing shoes too small. Genetics are responsible for a significant percentage of cases. Researchers have found bunions in people throughout the world who have never worn shoes.

WHEN TO STOP TRAINING

- The common sense guidelines apply to these injuries. Swelling, redness, inability to stride normally, increasing pain, and pain with daily activity—all are reasons to rest.

CONSEQUENCES OF RUNNING OR WALKING THROUGH THE PAIN

- Athletes often wait too long to seek help. The pain may be intermittent and not severe, often occurring only during longer workouts. The fear of surgery may also cause a delay in diagnosis. Unfortunately this denial allows a slow progression of changes to the bones and possibly permanent damage to the joint surfaces when they might have been treated. At this point, the only alternative may be surgery.

- There is a small but real risk of permanent damage by pushing through a single episode of pain. Sometimes the pain begins a few days before an important race. Realistically it may be worth the risk to attempt the race but be prepared to drop out if the pain becomes strong.

OUTSIDE OF FOOT—MIDWAY ON THE PROMINENT BONE

FIFTH METATARSAL STYLOID PROCESS INJURIES

LOCATION

- Outside of the foot midway on the prominent bone that is the rear of the fifth metatarsal bone.

- The tendon that prevents ankle sprains and raises the outside of the foot connects in this area. This tendon is the extension of the muscle in the outer leg and also helps the foot at push-off.

- Pain can be anywhere on the bony prominence or just ahead of it.

DESCRIPTION OF PAIN

- If the pain gradually increases in the back portion of the bone, hurts moderately with exercise and does not affect daily walking activity, this condition is usually "insertional tendinitis." This is the result of the tendon pulling hard away from the bone. Some people are born with an extra bone at this spot which becomes disturbed. The presence of the bone is a problem only when it becomes aggravated.

- Similar pain in this area that begins with an ankle sprain is also insertional tendinitis, but can involve a tear of the tendon from the bone, sometimes pulling a piece of bone away with the tendon. This can happen with surprisingly little pain, and can heal on its own.

- Pain involving the entire bony prominence or the front portion should be evaluated by a doctor.

- Stronger pain anywhere along the outside middle of the foot should also be analyzed because of the risk of the bone not healing. Stress fractures can progress to true fractures in this area very easily.

BASIC ANATOMY

- Tendons that attach in this area pull in different directions. When the muscles that attach to the tendons tighten, the fracture can open further and can even be a cause of the injury. So if there is even a tiny fracture, there is a very high probability that the break may not heal unless the injury is cared for properly. A couple of millimeters difference in location of the break can force one to put no weight on the foot at all.

- This area of the foot must tolerate strong forces. It is especially overloaded when the foot is supinated or when running on uneven surfaces for a long period of time.

- Some people have a naturally large shape to the bone, which can be easily irritated by shoes pressing or rubbing. Ski boots, tight dress shoes, and running shoes that are too narrow often cause pressure problems. This should be considered before assuming the injury is more serious.

CAUSES

- Too much supination puts pressure on the outside of the foot and is a common cause. When a new pair of shoes has too much correction, the following pattern can occur: The muscle whose tendon attaches to this spot is working on every step to lift the outside of the foot so it will straighten and is overused. The same thing happens when midsole or heels are too worn, tilting the foot to the outside (even slightly) with each step.

- An ankle sprain (when the foot rolls under) can cause pain in this area and may result in a complete fracture. In many cases the ankle itself is barely injured, the pain comes mostly from the foot.

TREATMENT

- Mild pain that begins gradually can be treated with ice, decreased mileage, or rest, and often from shifting to a less stable, more neutral shoe. Avoiding uneven surfaces and eliminating faster workouts can allow continuation of training as the injury heals.

- Evaluate your shoes. Any new shoe may be the cause including everyday shoes. Too narrow, too stable, or too worn shoes can be suspect.

- Strong pain, swelling, loss of function or pain that hurts to walk should be evaluated by a doctor.

PEARLS

- The "Jones Fracture" is a more serious stress fracture than I usually seen. It heals slowly and sometimes not at all without surgery. Make sure that the doctor that evaluates the foot can rule this out. Some doctors call all stress fractures "Jones Fractures," but this term should only be applied to this more troublesome, uncommon condition that should be treated immediately.

WHEN TO STOP TRAINING

- It is always better to take two to three days off of running if you suspect this injury. Also, don't finish a run if you may have this condition. Pain that persists through a run, and hurts a lot worse afterward, or causes pain on every walking step in your daily activities, indicates a need for rest and treatment.

- Stronger pain should be evaluated by a doctor. Stop running to keep from making the injury worse.

CONSEQUENCES OF RUNNING OR WALKING THROUGH THE PAIN

- Running with mild pain, mentioned above, is normal.

- Aggravating a stress reaction into a true fracture is easily done in this area by running with pain.

- If the injury progresses it can take months to heal and may require surgery.

OUTER SIDE OF HEEL—ALSO BELOW ANKLE BONE MOVING TOWARD MIDFOOT ON OUTSIDE

PERONEAL TENDON INJURY OUTER HEEL AREA AND CUBOID SYNDROME

LOCATION

- Outer side of the heel and just forward of the heel bone.

- Below ankle bone as far forward (on the outside of the foot) as the base of the fifth metatarsal styloid process and as far back as directly below the back edge of the ankle bone.

- Pain is usually on the side, but sometimes is felt on the bottom of the foot in the same area.

DESCRIPTION OF PAIN

- A general achy feeling.

- Comes on gradually and a specific place is sometimes difficult to locate.

- Usually present with everyday walking.

- Usually the pain does not prevent running/walking. But after a workout, the foot may be sore. At the beginning, the area may be sore and may take a few minutes to warm up.

- Sharper, more intense pain indicates another injury—especially if pain comes from deep inside the foot or ankle.

- Pain in this area after a mild ankle sprain is normal. If you suffered a painful sprain, have a doctor look into this.

BASIC ANATOMY

- The peroneal tendons run from the back of the bottom of the outer ankle bone to the styloid process of the fifth metatarsal and just behind the fifth metatarsal, wrapping under the outside of the foot.

- The pain does not need to be reproduced along this tendon by touching to indicate this injury.

- Sometimes the ligaments that connect the cuboid bone to the others become irritated or injured. This bone is the high point of what is called the lateral arch and it receives significant stress when running. The sensation is similar to a sprain.

- Pain reproduced at the tip of the ankle bone is not this injury.

CAUSES

- Many shoes are too soft at the outer heel. This allows the heel to tilt and the extra motion aggravates the area.

- Wearing certain types of casual/work (nonrunning) shoes can also be a cause if they tilt the heel—and wearing sandals.

- Changing from a worn and broken-in shoe to a stiffer, new shoe can be a cause. Any change in shoes should be investigated.

- Wearing new orthotics (medical or over-the-counter types) can be a cause, especially if the new device is too angled. While it is common to experience this feeling (in a mild way) for a day or two as you break in a new pair, this should go away.

- When a runner who pronates heavily is given a shoe that offers too much correction, this problem can be produced, especially if there has been no problem when wearing a more neutral shoe. The anti-pronation shoes raise the inside of the foot so that suddenly the lateral arch is supporting the weight and forcing the foot to move more to the outside at push-off. Unfortunately the ligaments that hold the cuboid bone in position are not adequately conditioned and a painful stretching can occur. If the adaptation to the more rigid foot position could occur more gradually, this situation can be avoided, allowing for a transition from pronation to occur.

TREATMENT

- Shoes with more lateral firmness and stability will gradually allow the injury to heal, usually while continuing to work out.

- Sometimes a comfortable ankle support that can be purchased at running or drug stores can speed the healing process.

- When the cuboid bone is involved, foot taping may help; see a qualified physical trainer, physical therapist or podiatrist.

- Soft support under the cuboid bone may help, but not if the area is too tender.

- Serious cases may need orthotics.

- If the pain progresses, or lasts more than five or six weeks, see a doctor.

- If the pain was caused by a change of shoes, return to the older style until the injury heals.

PEARLS

- Try to feel the tendons (often they are very small and hard to find). If they are tender and swollen, see a doctor.

- This injury is one that occurs often, responds well to changing the tilt of the foot, and is often mistaken for other injuries. Once treatment has begun, it may take a few days to see improvement if training continues. Running/ walking while the injury is healing is possible and typical as long as the guidelines are followed.

- Cuboid Syndrome has traditionally been treated with a form of foot manipulation. Years of experience have shown that this is rarely helpful and sometimes makes it worse. Often this treatment is performed along with taping and other forms of therapy which is what enhances the healing process.

WHEN TO STOP TRAINING

- If the pain is ever sharp, piercing, or if swelling is noted, stop training and see a doctor.

CONSEQUENCES OF RUNNING OR WALKING THROUGH THE PAIN

- Recovery will take a little longer without rest, but it should improve steadily.

- Other injuries in this location can be more serious including stress fractures and torn tendons. If there is any possibility of these other conditions, see a doctor immediately.

INSIDE OF FOOT AT ANKLE BONE

TIBIALIS POSTERIOR MEDIAL FOOT/TARSAL TUNNEL

LOCATION OF PAIN

- The pain is noticed along the inside of the foot at the ankle bone running forward for an inch or two. It can be located anywhere in this region.

- In many cases the pain is experienced only on the inside of the foot halfway forward. Another site may be near the ankle bone. Pain will often be in a specific area.

- Pain may also travel underneath the inside of the foot and feel very deep.

- Sometimes this condition may be mistaken for a sore inner ankle bone.

DESCRIPTION OF PAIN

- At first, there is a gradual increase in pain, starting during a single run/walk. A sudden increase in pain in this area often indicates a more serious injury.

- If the pain began as an ankle sprain, it is not this injury.

- The sensation is more of an achiness with general soreness. Again, if there is sharp pain, see a doctor.

- It is felt when the foot is flat and pushing off.

- Mild cases can be relieved by walking on the outside of the foot. But eventually, this will not help because the injured tendon is working very hard to hold the foot on the outer edge. This will cause the injury to progress.

- Rest allows the pain to diminish, but everyday walking can bring it back.

- Sometimes cramping or muscle spasm may occur along the inside of the foot or just underneath the inside. This may be at night or when weight is off the foot for a few minutes.

BASIC ANATOMY

- Pain comes from a very important tendon that begins as a muscle on the inside of the leg, travels behind the inner ankle bone and attaches to the inner side of the foot and slightly underneath the inner foot. This muscle and tendon supports the arch and lifts the inside of the foot to prevent excessive pronation and to help with propulsion.

- There are two additional tendons, a vein, an artery, and a nerve that pass through a narrow tunnel with this tendon. They are held in place by a tight strap of tough tissue which pushes against these structures when the heel rolls inward and the arch flattens excessively.

- The other two tendons also assist in lifting the arch, as they curl the toes downward. They can also be injured and produce very similar pain. When these tendons are injured through running or walking, the same initial treatment is used. A doctor would need to locate which tendon is involved and the damage site before extensive treatment is performed.

- Sometimes the nerve is also irritated. This is commonly called tarsal tunnel syndrome. In this case, the pain radiates from under the foot. This injury is often misdiagnosed. In many cases the pain emanates from the plantar fascia that also supports the arch. The plantar fascia is often sore at the same time because foot types that have extra stress on the tibialis posterior tendon are also likely to have more stress on the plantar fascia.

- If a tendon in the tunnel is injured, it will be thicker. This can put pressure on the nerve, which if significant enough, may cause pain or unusual sensations such as tingling or decreased feeling. Usually, after the tendon heals, all of the nerve problems go away, but this may take a while longer since nerves take longer to recover.

CAUSES

- Low arched feet are more likely to stress the tendons in this area.

- Excessive pronation (foot rolls to the inside as it pushes off).

- Wearing shoes that do not have enough stability to match the motion of the foot (it may take weeks before pain is experienced due to shoe choice).

- Everyday shoes that have little or no support: flip-flops, women's flats.

- Walking barefooted.

- Wearing racing flats instead of supportive running shoes.

- Extended run/walk on a slanted surface such as a side of a road.

TREATMENT

- Initial treatment usually starts with a significant increase in arch support to prevent or reduce pronation. It helps to use more stable (motion control or stability) running shoes, over-the-counter orthotics, arch taping. Don't walk barefoot, and don't use unstable everyday shoes. These adjustments will often allow for running while the healing is proceeding.

- Icing is helpful for recovery and usually reduces the duration of the injury. For 15 minutes every night, rub a chunk of ice directly on the injured area until it gets numb.

- Elastic ankle supports may help, but are not as good as stable running shoes with orthotic arch supports. The compression and guidance of an ankle support helps with everyday activities and very mild injuries, however. For maximum support use all of the above.

- If there is soreness or swelling in the tendon which runs from the bottom of the ankle bone to the bony inner side of the foot, avoid running for at least three days. Injuries that produce mild soreness usually respond to the above-mentioned self-treatment. But when there is swelling and strong pain, see a doctor. The tibialis posterior tendon is vital to running and walking. A tearing or rupture of this tendon can lead to a fallen arch, arthritis, and often extensive surgery.

- Physical therapy is helpful, but avoid strengthening exercises until the injury is healing successfully. It is difficult to strengthen the tibialis posterior muscle to the extent that it can overcome an inferior inherited foot structure. Long-term strengthening of the feet is very important to decrease the likelihood of reinjury.

- A doctor may also prescribe immobilization with a cast or removable walker. This is advised if the injury is not healing and training is not possible. Gentle activities or non weight bearing motion with crutches is also a possibility.

- A doctor may prescribe an MRI to see if there is a tear or to identify which tendon is injured. This can be helpful if a more aggressive treatment is needed.

- Do not allow an injection directly to the tibialis posterior tendon unless everything else has failed, months of rest have not produced healing, and there is the possibility of a rupture. The other two tendons in this area are less risky to inject, but still pose risks. Again, an MRI may determine the location of the damage.

- If a nerve conduction study is recommended (for possible tarsal tunnel nerve symptoms) try to find a specialist that has worked with a lot of runners in this area. A positive result from this test may mean the nerve is damaged, but there is no standard treatment when this happens. Surgery will not heal the nerve if it is significantly injured and it usually will not show as a positive study unless it is. The nerve can be injured even when the results say "normal." Be sure that your doctor is doing a thorough job of conservative treatment to allow sufficient time for healing to occur.

- Medical custom orthotics are needed if the pain is recurrent, or if the injury is due to poor foot structure, rather than training or shoe errors.

PEARLS

- If very thorough support with good shoes does not seem to be promoting healing, you could have a tear.

- Mild to moderate cases heal very quickly—usually within a couple of weeks.

- When the tendon is significantly injured, healing can take three to four months.

- If a true tibialis posterior tendon tear (not a rupture) has happened, six months to a full year off from running is usually necessary in order to avoid surgery. Choose alternative exercise carefully.

- If the tendon is ruptured or stretched (attenuated is the medical term), surgery is usually recommended and long distance running sports may not be possible.

WHEN TO STOP TRAINING

- Most of the time it is possible to continue training when damage is minor. Common sense dictates that the possibility of tearing a tendon increases greatly if it is already swollen and sore. So if there is inflammation or strong pain, stop running and see a doctor.

CONSEQUENCES OF RUNNING OR WALKING THROUGH PAIN

- A tear may result in a collapsed ankle and/or foot.

- Significant damage may reduce ability to push off or stride normally, and can cause more severe injuries in the hamstring and other areas, due to compensation.

BOTTOM OF HEEL (OFTEN INSIDE)—MAY EXTEND ALONG BOTTOM OF ARCH TO FRONT OF FOOT

PLANTAR FASCIITIS

LOCATION

- Can include any or all of these locations:

  1. Bottom of the heel with possibly radiating pain up the sides.

  2. Back of the heel.

  3. The arch on the underside of the foot from the heel forward to the ball of the foot.

  4. Very commonly it is felt on the inside of the heel, moving toward the arch area.

DESCRIPTION OF PAIN

- Plantar fascia pain is first noticed on the bottom of the heel. It may also hurt on the underside of the foot in the arch or both locations at once. Pain after sitting or sleeping is characteristic especially when taking the first few steps in the morning. Usually the pain increases with lots of activity, but it will often warm up and decrease after a few minutes when walking or running. More severe cases will not warm up and may literally cause a person to limp. Milder cases may remain only slightly annoying and decrease with days of rest, only to return after a few days of training again.

BASIC ANATOMY

- The plantar fascia is a tough flat strap of connective tissue that attaches to the bottom and forward part of the underside of the heel. It fans out to the ball of the foot. When you bend your toes up, you can feel the central slip of the band tighten and appear at the back of the arch near the heel. There are two other slips, one fans to the inner side of the arch and one runs to the outside of the arch near the bottom of the bone halfway up the outside of the foot (styloid process of the fifth metatarsal). Most injuries involve stretching or tearing of a few of the fibers in this band anywhere from the heel bone forward.

- Serious cases can involve a complete tear of this area and the band may become loose and no longer tighten as is normal. The purpose of the plantar fascia is to support the curved shape of the arch of the foot. If the fascia was absent the foot would no longer be a rigid structure at push-off. When it is inadequate, the foot remains loose and lacks spring which can cause overload of other joints. It is extremely rare that a plantar fascia injury causes a noticeable loss of arch height, although a mild fallen arch can occur. The tissue has a poor ability to repair itself because it is fibrous connective tissue lacking abundant blood flow. It can also pull away from the heel and cause true damage to the surface of the bone. Sometimes as it heals, a thickened area will temporarily form as repair tissue tries to bridge the weakened defect. If this tissue appears on the bottom of the heel, it can be mistaken for a heel spur. Some doctors call it bursitis, but it is not a true bursitis. Heel spurs can form at this junction, but spurs are unlikely to be a cause of pain. They nearly always are far above the surface we stand on. Heel spurs appear in many people who have never had heel pain, and we believe the spur is just a collection of calcium that is formed when inflammation is present. In some people the calcium can become so concentrated that it no longer can stay in solution and collects along the fibers of the fascia as in the formation of a crystal. There is no direct correlation with the presence of a spur and the amount of pain or recurrence.

CAUSES

- The injury of the fascia occurs when the force downward on the arch stretches the fascia beyond its strength. Singular episodes may produce this, but it is much more common to appear gradually. Running in old or poorly supporting shoes, too much time or too quick of a transition to racing flats or spikes may be a cause. But it is often aggravated by the shoes worn when not running. Walking too long in sandals or barefoot, weight gain, and overdoing other activities (such as jump rope, dance, and weight lifting) are prime causes. PF can occur in any type of foot and is not more likely to occur in flat feet.

TREATMENT

- Initial treatment is focused on supporting the arch to prevent the stretching force—even for pain on the bottom of the heel. Although heel padding may feel better initially, because of the tender heel, true healing is best achieved with proper support of the arch, as soon as the PF is diagnosed.

- Wear supportive shoes at all times – especially when stepping out of bed in the morning.

- Purchase over-the-counter orthotics (arch supports).

- Tape the foot using the arch support method. Leave the tape on as much as possible.

- Ice the sore area for 20 minutes daily and when it becomes extra sore, use the ice massage method.

- If pain progresses beyond 2 to 3 weeks, add these treatments:

- Use a night splint for sleeping (best to get advice from a podiatrist before doing this).

- Begin a gentle calf stretching program (get advice first and be very, very gentle if you do this).

- Carefully begin daily arch massage (tennis ball, small frozen water filled bottle).

- If improvement is slow or nonexistent, and one is unable to run/walk after four to six weeks:

- See a doctor (best if this is someone who specializes in foot problems for athletes).

- Consider custom medical orthotics made by an experienced person.

PEARLS

- Do not stretch the arch itself, especially in the first couple of months.

- Do not have a cortisone injection unless orthotics, taping, and rest have failed to provide adequate relief. This can weaken the fascia and result in further damage if the foot is not protected for an extended period of time after the injection. Cortisone artificially blocks the pain and many PF victims increase the damage without knowing it during the painless period. In most cases, if used correctly and carefully, an injection can be a valuable treatment for serious cases.

- Mild cases may heal in a few weeks to a couple of months, but it is common for a serious injury to last a year before completely disappearing. During this time it is normal to have mild ache and a slightly sensitive heel or arch. You should be able to run/walk with no pain after a short warm-up and only mild stiffness later. Orthotics and supportive shoes can prevent pain during the recovery. If the pain is within these parameters, the healing is progressing normally and should disappear gradually. If you are unable to run/walk without strong pain or if the pain is not almost gone at 12 months, further medical treatment should be considered.

- Surgery is prescribed too often. It is an easy procedure and some doctors are eager to perform it. This involves cutting the fascia two-thirds across, lengthening the fascia and reducing the tension. While this can work, I see a lot of patients who did not experience relief. Even when it works for the original fascia injury, losing the normal strength and length of the fascia can result in secondary problems throughout the foot, often experienced months later.

- Many doctors are sidetracked by the "diagnosis of the month." Pain on the outside of the heel is confused with a nerve entrapment. Pain on the inner side of the heel is thought to be tarsal tunnel syndrome. These conditions are extremely rare and thousands of dollars have been wasted on expensive diagnostic and treatment modalities. Plantar fascia pain is variable and inconsistent and if the original fascia injury heals properly, the nearby pains nearly always go away. If you are told you have another more rare condition, be very skeptical and perhaps consider a second opinion.

- Plantar fasciitis is rare in people with strong feet.

WHEN TO STOP TRAINING

- It is wise to take a few days off at the earliest sign of any injury. If the damage caused by the initial injury is very substantial, rest will not cure the problem in a few days to a couple of weeks. In this case it is necessary to search for other ways to keep running while healing the injury.

- Until the tissue fully heals it is OK to run with mild pain as described in PEARLS section above, but it is not wise to run through stronger pain.

- It is best to avoid speedwork, fast running and hill training when there is significant pain in the PF.

CONSEQUENCES OF RUNNING OR WALKING THROUGH THE PAIN

- Pain beyond the mild category may indicate continued progression of damage to the fascia and heel. This means it will take longer to heal.

- People who completely push through the pain often need two or three years to heal.

- People who follow the guidelines mentioned above and are careful to keep the pain in the mild category, heal very well while continuing to run.

PREVENTION

- Jeff has had great success with his runners in preventing PF by using what he calls the "toe squincher" exercise: point your foot down and contract the muscles in the foot until they cramp. You can do this 10 to 20 times with each foot, per day.

BACK OF HEEL, SOMETIMES UNDERNEATH

POSTERIOR HEEL PAIN

LOCATION OF PAIN

- The pain from this condition is usually experienced on the back of the heel and even partially underneath it. In some cases, sensation may fan onto either or both sides of the heel. It usually extends up the back of the heel but not in every case. Pain in the Achilles tendon above the heel is discussed in the ankle injury section, but is indirectly related to this injury.

DESCRIPTION OF PAIN

- Pain can vary from a dull ache to a sharp, piercing sensation.

- Only in severe cases does it hurt when not standing, walking, or running.

- In most cases, only one foot is affected. The main exception is growth center pain in children and teenagers.

- Swelling can occur higher on the back of the heel.

- It is common to feel this during the first few steps in the morning, and during the first few minutes of running or walking, and then have it go away during the workout.

BASIC ANATOMY

- The Achilles tendon is an extension of the calf muscles, and inserts into the back of the heel. It fans out across the entire width of the heel. Only the deepest fibers of the tendon attach directly to the heel bone. The others continue around the bottom of the heel and become the plantar fascia. So while it is attached to the lower half of the heel directly to the bone, it acts as a strap that wraps around the bottom.

- There is a layer of connective tissue that contains fluid, called a bursa, between the tendon and the upper third of the back of the heel—above the attachment of the tendon to the heel bone.

- Those with high arches often have a bump high on the back of the heel. The high arch condition forces the heel bone to be tilted backward into the Achilles tendon, forcing the uppermost portion of the back of the heel bone to rub against the tendon. Eventually, due to constant irritation, a bony protrusion develops. This is called a Haglund's deformity. While commonly occurring, this can rub more easily on the tendon, irritating it due to pressure from the shoe. This often inflames the bursa which produces redness and swelling associated with Haglund's deformity. Long-term excessive rubbing on the bone can cause continuous growth of the bump and it can become a very large, easily irritated protrusion.

- Those with high arches are more prone to Haglund's deformity and likely to supinate with heels that move at an angle. This outward tilt on the heel will produce a stronger rubbing on the outer portion of the Achilles tendon insertion. The size of the bump on the outer corner will often increase in this case, and is troublesome because it focuses more force on a smaller area. Bone spurs where the tendon connects can also result.

- Those with low arches and no posterior bump can also experience pain in this area, which usually heals more easily.

- The Achilles tendon can be torn where it wraps onto the heel if it is irritated excessively.

- Pain on the lowest part of the back of the heel is a variant of plantar fasciitis. The location of injury is slightly different, but some of the plantar fascia treatments are effective (see the section in this book).

- Children and teenagers have a softer layer of cartilage in the heel bone that is a growth center. Long bones have this type of growth center called an apophysis: heel, legs, fingers, and arms—unlike flat bones like the skull. It provides a more rapidly reproducing supply of cells than regular bone cells. As they mature, these cells turn into bone, lengthening the bone due to the speed of reproduction. The Achilles tendon attaches to the back of the heel, near the apophysis, and the plantar fascia attaches near the apophysis on the bottom of the heel. The significant pull between these two structures can irritate the softer material of the apophysis, resulting in calcaneal apophysitis or Sever's disease. Repetitive motion and irritation of the heel apophysis does not affect the growth or outcome of the heel bone as an adult.

CAUSES

- Pain in the back of the heel is most commonly insertional Achilles tendinitis. This can be due to irritation of the bursa, the tendon fibers, or the heel bone, usually caused by the powerful force of the Achilles tendon. Those who develop posterior heel pain usually have a flaw in the foot that focuses extra pressure and can cause injury in this area.

- Excessive pronation or supination can produce extra stress on a portion of the tendon due to the foot turning outward or inward, repetitively.

- Various forms of arthritis cause heel pain—most commonly among those who have arthritis in other parts of the body.

- Heel pain in children and teenagers (mentioned previously) can result from any sport that requires running. Higher arches, greater impact, and overuse are causes. Children have the energy and power to overuse orthopedic units, anywhere—regardless of foot type.

- Stretching the Achilles tendon too strongly or too often is commonly a cause of lower posterior heel pain. Running or walking on soft surfaces such as sand or snow, and jumping drills (jump rope) can also produce this injury.

- Pressure on the back of the heel can result in bursitis. Common causes are wearing shoes that are too short, spending hours in rigid boots (such as ski boots), and sitting for long periods with heels resting on a firm surface.

TREATMENT

- Icing is very useful for this injury. Use a chunk of ice, rubbed constantly and directly on the area for 15 minutes every evening.

- Don't ignore the pain. Low-intensity pain is easy to tolerate, but running with this injury will usually make it much worse and greatly lengthen the recovery time needed.

- Heel lifts should be worn in all shoes. High heels or shoes with more than a moderate heel height can aggravate the injured areas.

- Walking is much better tolerated than running, and can maintain most of the adaptations when normal distances are covered.

- Proper shoe choice, aided by knowledgeable running store staff can reduce pronation or supination.

- Sometimes off-the-shelf orthotics or softer orthotics can help. But if these do not seem to result in quicker healing, custom orthotics can produce a better result, over a longer time period. Ask your doctor.

- Avoid hills and speed workouts!

- For apophysitis (bony protuberance), a padded heel cup, available at many running stores, may cure the problem. If not, supportive arch taping and a good off-the-shelf orthotic may reduce irritation so that healing can proceed. Only in a rare case is a custom orthotic necessary.

- Sometimes these initial treatments do not help. A doctor will probably x-ray the heel to see if there is a spur, based upon evidence of protrusion. The presence of this bony mass makes it more difficult to heal and more susceptible to injury, but removal is not often necessary. Many people have them and never develop pain. A doctor can tell by examination whether a bursa irritation is suspected. Sometimes an MRI exam is useful if the pain continues with little or no healing to identify if the bursa is inflamed, the bone injured, or the tendon damaged. Treatment will target which area is damaged. Injections should be avoided in this area due to the risk of Achilles tendon rupture. If all other treatments have failed, and the injury has been present for months, an injection directed deep to the tendon and confined to the bursa can sometimes work. In this case, stop running and look into wearing a cast or boot for about a month.

- Surgery to repair the heel can be an option in extreme cases. There is no guarantee of success, and there are several procedures. Lateral Haglund's bump removal, above the tendon insertion, is quite effective and relatively simple. This requires at least eight weeks of nonrunning recovery time. The surgery will not be a cure if the bump is not the problem. When considering surgery, try to find an experienced doctor, and ask for a thorough diagnosis. In some cases, the tendon is detached and then reattached with bone anchors.

- Physical therapy, acupuncture, and other adjunctive treatments may be helpful. Laser, ultrasound, iontophoresis, phonophoresis, electrical, ultramagnetic, and topical treatments have had a certain percentage of success. Recently there have been good reports about high intensity ultrasound shock-wave therapy. This is called ESWT. There is also a newer form of lower intensity therapy and the initial reports have been very good. While not all types of injuries respond, a number of surgeries are avoided and injuries managed by using this treatment. A good diagnosis is important when the injury is advanced.

- This injury may require weeks of immobilization to heal.

- As a last resort, if surgery is the only remaining option, six months of no running is recommended. This choice is difficult. Certain variations of posterior heel pain take a long time to heal and will only do so if there is no significant irritation to the area. If such a rest period has been taken, and pain is still present, surgery is an option.

- For apophysitis in children and teenagers, a padded heel cup, purchased at a running store, may cure the problem. If not, supportive arch taping and off-the-shelf orthotics may speed the healing process. In rare cases, custom orthotics are necessary. Children outgrow them quickly so for practical reasons, off-the-shelf devices are recommended. The growth centers remain open until the age of 16 or 17 years for boys and around 15 for girls. Luckily the apophysis does not have to close completely to have the pain disappear. If there is heel pain in those older than this, it is not apophysitis.

PEARLS

- Many people need to use heel lifts (in shoes) permanently, to prevent recurrent problems.

- Stretching the Achilles tendon during a period of acute pain will probably make the condition worse. Sometimes a night splint can help, so have a doctor look carefully at this as a treatment mode. Note that there is a sock device that is sometimes prescribed for plantar fasciitis that does not work very well for this posterior heel problem. Overdoing a night splint is possible, so be careful.

- It is important to keep the heel as straight as possible in running and walking. Custom orthotics may require a couple of experimental modifications to find the optimal position—but they can produce successful results. Making adjustments to orthotics is a normal part of the process, and not a reflection of poor understanding by the doctor. In many cases, the first versions may overcorrect temporarily, but can be modified to work, and gradually reduce the correction, as the injury heals.

- Many great athletes have had to retire from competition because of severe posterior heel damage. It is important to address the problem early.

WHEN TO STOP TRAINING

- Early rest can prevent long-term complications. Remember, a high percentage of these injuries are caused by the bursa becoming inflamed. When the bursa is sore, it becomes enlarged and attracts a fluid buildup. That increases pressure on the area. So, activity accelerates the swelling and damage. Resting for a few days may allow the swelling to decrease while you continue to work out gently as the bursa shrinks.

CONSEQUENCES OF RUNNING OR WALKING THROUGH PAIN

- A single episode of pain may heal quickly and cause no further problems. If the pain appears during an important race and rest afterward is planned, it is logical to continue.

- Continuing to train with pain for a long time is a poor idea because permanent growth of the heel bone bump or spur occurs. Permanent damage to the tendon is possible and the bursa can develop fibrotic scarring and never shrink back to its normal size.

THE ANKLE

OUTSIDE OF THE ANKLE MOSTLY BUT CAN BE ON THE INSIDE

ANKLE SPRAINS

LOCATION OF PAIN

- Pain is generated around the outer ankle when the foot rolls excessively to the outside. This is called an inversion sprain.

- Less commonly, the inner ankle is injured (an eversion strain) when the foot rolls too far to the inside.

- The primary areas affected by an inversion sprain are the ankle bone, the leg, or on the top of the foot.

- Eversion sprains produce pain around the inner ankle bone/inner side of the foot. Occasionally pain is experienced in the area just above the ankle.

- Sprains can produce damage in other areas of the leg and foot. If you're experiencing unusual pain in an unexpected area it should be evaluated.

TYPES OF ANKLE SPRAINS

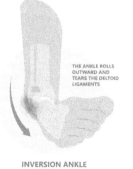
THE ANKLE ROLLS OUTWARD AND TEARS THE DELTOID LIGAMENTS

INVERSION ANKLE SPRAINS

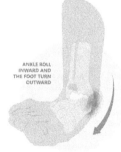
ANKLE ROLL INWARD AND THE FOOT TURN OUTWARD

EVERSION ANKLE SPRAINS

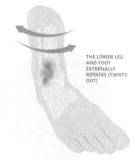
THE LOWER LEG AND FOOT EXTERNALLY ROTATES (TWISTS OUT)

HIGH ANKLE SPRAINS

BASIC ANATOMY

- Three ligaments attach the outer ankle bone to the foot. During a normal running/walking motion, the foot rolls to a neutral position, and the ankle balances the forces of bodyweight and forward movement. When the foot continues to roll excessively, the primary ligaments are severely stressed and can tear. It is not uncommon for the stress on the bone to be so great, where the ligaments connect, that the bone will break. The torque of the foot as it rolls over the bones creates enough stress to fracture bones far from the ligaments. Sometimes the ligaments at the ankle are spared and the only effect is sore tendons.

- Eversion sprains can injure the large sturdy ligament around the inner ankle bone or pull the tendons that support the arch, originating on the inner leg and ankle. An injury to the large inner ankle ligament can take a long time to heal.

CAUSES

- Inversion sprains are usually the result of running on an unexpected, irregular surface. Those with weak ankles are more prone. Unstable shoes also increase risk.

- Eversion sprains are also experienced by those running/walking on unstable surfaces. Those who are heavier, who have weak ankles and who pronate add stress and increase risk.

- There are far more eversion sprains produced in lateral movement sports (soccer, football, basketball) than in linear sports like running/walking.

TREATMENT

- Initially, get a good evaluation of the ankle. In most cases, the incident occurs in the middle of a workout and the runner/walker must find a way to get back to home. The body is designed to keep you moving forward for a few minutes with minimal pain—even when the sprain is fairly serious. Movement is not possible when there is a serious sprain or a fracture, and fortunately these are uncommon. At the moment of injury, it is very difficult to interpret the damage unless the sprain was severe. Even when the ankle "pops," the injury is not always severe as in a broken bone. Most commonly the sound is due to the ankle being stretched so that the highest foot bone leans out of its tight-fitting socket. The pop can be the suction being released.

- Sometimes the act of running/walking (if possible) can pump blood and fluid so that the pain is reduced or gradually goes away. It is very unlikely that continuing for a short distance will cause further damage as long as the pain remains mild, and the foot/leg is working somewhat normally.

- If pain is sharp, or forces one to limp, it is possible to carefully and gently continue to the next stopping point. If the sprain happened while running, shift to walking.

- If the pain rapidly increases with each step, it is wise to stop and get help.

- If you cannot support yourself or the pain is intense, get help immediately and consider treatment for shock as well.

- Immediate compression should be applied even for minor sprains: elastic compression sleeve, wrap with elastic wrap, etc.

- Apply ice immediately. Pack the wrapped ankle with ice and elevate the foot above the head if possible.

- In severe cases, it is best to see a doctor quickly (emergency room). If surgery is needed, the best timing is before swelling occurs. Otherwise there may be a significant delay in treatment to allow for the inflammation to go away.

- After the first hour or two of compression and ice, continue to use compression as noted, and ice for 20 minutes, every 2 to 3 hours. By preventing significant inflammation, you will speed the healing. After a few days, the elastic tape can usually be terminated but an elastic ankle sleeve is recommended.

- See a doctor as soon as you can IF 1) the swelling is quite noticeable despite these treatments, 2) you cannot support body weight, or 3) the pain remains strong.

- A doctor will take an x-ray to see whether you have a fracture. Some ankle fractures do not hurt as much as would be expected, some do not require a cast and walking might be possible. Physical therapy may be recommended, and this can speed the recovery.

- If the sprain is mild enough to treat at home, it is wise to avoid exercise until the swelling has almost disappeared and there is no pain when walking. A test run/walk of 20 minutes will determine if training can begin. On your first few runs it's best to insert a 10- to 15-second run break into each minute of walking. It is usually safe to exercise if mild soreness appears, but if there is swelling, pain that is noticeable, there is a significant change in foot plant or stride, or the soreness continues into daily walking, workouts should be delayed. Wait a couple of days and try again.

- Most inversion sprains that are safe to treat at home heal in less than three to four weeks with an average term of two weeks. Eversion sprains often require an average of two more weeks.

- It is wise to consider a small elastic ankle brace when restarting your workouts. During the first few weeks of healing, there is a greater risk of another sprain because the tendons and sensory nerves are disturbed and reaction times are slower. The brace will help the ankle react to sudden forces more quickly and decrease the possibility of rolling it again.

- Eversion sprains are more serious, and if there is swelling, limping, and pain, see a doctor. If it hurts moderately without swelling, use the same icing and treatment as with inversion sprains. It also helps to prevent pronation or allow the foot to have a slight supination during recovery from an eversion sprain, because the inside of the ankle must work hard with every step. The workload is less when pronation is eliminated.

PROPRIOCEPTION EXERCISES FOR REHAB AND TO PREVENT FUTURE SPRAINS

These exercises train the nerves and rapidly firing muscles to adapt to uneven terrain to prevent future sprains. When these exercises do not cause a pain flair up, it is safe to try test workouts. Even after you have restarted your training, it's best to continue the exercises for a few weeks. Unless the injury prevented activity for several weeks, general strengthening exercises are not as important as these. Overall ankle strength will improve as training resumes. Strengthening the ankle is recommended for recurrent sprains, after a cast or immobilization, or tendon injuries.

- As soon as the pain has decreased, begin treatment as you prepare for a return to activity. While sitting with the foot elevated, bend the ankle up and down. Point the toes downward and then upward over and over for about a minute. A small amount of mild pain is normal—but take an extra rest day if pain is sharp or strong. This exercise can be done many times each day if you are not increasing the aggravation.

- When there is no pain during the exercise above, a second stage can be added: While sitting with the foot elevated as before, imagine that the tip of the big toe is the point of a pencil. Hold the leg still but rotate the ankle while writing the alphabet with the end of the toes. This rotation exercise can be performed many times a day.

- When no pain is experienced with the previous exercise, begin standing exercises. The most convenient and effective ones are simple and require no equipment. Stand on the injured leg and balance on the foot. Raise the uninjured leg off of the ground and swing it from side to side both in front and behind, rapidly changing directions for one minute. This requires good balance. If unable to perform this without touching, repeat this until you are able to reach one minute almost every time. Don't use your hands and arms for balance. Wearing shoes is suggested.

- Next, do this exercise barefooted eventually standing barefoot on a soft surface such as grass or a pillow. The final test is to perform it with the eyes closed.

PEARLS

- It is normal to feel nervous on irregular terrain for months after a sprain.

- It takes months for a torn ligament to completely repair itself. If the ankle is sprained repeatedly, the ligament may never heal.

WHEN TO STOP TRAINING

- No workouts should be considered if there is swelling or when you cannot run/walk with a normal stride. Mild pain can be expected when returning to workouts. There should be a reduction in the duration and intensity, however. If the improvement slows or stops, take more rest days.

CONSEQUENCES OF RUNNING OR WALKING THROUGH PAIN

- When an ankle is swollen and painful, it cannot protect the cartilage surfaces and tendons from stress. The body shifts to a healing/protection mode, and doesn't adapt to exercise until enough damage has been repaired. If the ankle is overused during this time, healing slows or stops, and more damage can be produced.

ON OR AROUND THE OUTER ANKLE BONE

OUTER ANKLE

LOCATION OF PAIN

- On or around the outer ankle bone.

- Pain on the outer leg bone (fibula) just above the large ankle bone or just behind it.

DESCRIPTION OF PAIN

- Pain caused by a fresh ankle sprain is not this injury.

- Leftover pain from an old ankle sprain is a reason for this injury. This type of pain is a soreness or ache that grows with activity. It may be very mild or nonexistent in everyday walking, but painful when aggravated by activity.

- Pain (without any ankle sprain incident) that often starts as a feeling of stiffness behind the ankle bone or a couple of inches higher.

- If it only hurts near the ankle bone, it can be mistaken for Achilles tendinitis unless the bone itself is sore.

- Sharp pain on the bone itself is possible and more of a concern.

BASIC ANATOMY

- There are three ligaments that connect the outer ankle bone to the foot. These are stretched and sometimes torn when an ankle is sprained. They may require a long time to mend enough to feel "normal," and sometimes never completely heal. As the foot bends at the ankle, the ligaments, when thickened or weakened from injury, are painfully stretched or sometimes pinched between the ankle bone and the foot.

- Sprains may also stretch and injure two tendons (peroneus longus and peroneus brevis) that originate from muscles in the outer leg. These muscles become tendons that travel together down the lower leg bone and through a groove in the back and bottom of the large ankle bone knob (lateral malleolus). When the ankle rolls over into inversion (to the outside), these tendons are often pulled beyond their normal length and damaged.

- Common tendinitis can develop in the two tendons (when grouped together, the peroneal tendons) and can progress from mild soreness to true tearing and rupture (extremely rare).

- The bone itself can develop a stress fracture. These are usually above the large ankle bone in the narrow portion of bone.

CAUSES

- Residual ankle sprain injuries can make this area vulnerable due to changes in the tissue caused by a sprain. Pronation that would not have caused the ankle bone to pinch the tendons, sheath, ligaments or joint capsule against the outer foot bones could be a problem after they became thicker from the sprain. Even mild excessive pronation can cause irritation near the prominent ankle bone, the malleolus.

- It is nearly always supination that causes classic gradual onset tendinitis of the peroneal tendons. Since they never get a chance to relax when the foot is supinated, they become irritated and inflamed. This can lead to more and more damage if neglected. In advanced cases, the tendons press against each other as they wrap under the sharp angle of the outer ankle bone (malleolus), and the narrow one may cut into the flatter one inducing a tear.

This can also happen during an ankle sprain, producing damage that does not allow continued training without significant increase in damage and pain.

- When these tendons do not fit tightly in the groove, they tend to extend onto the outer side of the ankle bone. This results in a sudden pain or feeling of the ankle "going out." Many people drop to the ground as if they had a sprain when this happens. Because the tendons return to the groove instantly, it is difficult for a nonmedical person to diagnose this.

- These problems can continue as a low grade irritation, and never develop into a serious condition. This mild form responds well to use of ice, new shoes, rest, decreased mileage, and an elastic ankle brace.

- If, after a sprain the injury seemed to heal during a layoff, pain increases around the ankle bone as training resumes, pronation is often a cause. Due to the original injury, the ankle components may have changed and more motion-controlling shoes may be needed.

- If no sprain is involved and pain begins around the ankle bone, the cause could be overpronation or excess supination, especially if there was a recent change in shoes or mileage. Get help from a good running shoe store or running form expert who can often identify whether pronation or supination could be a cause.

- If pain develops gradually from just above the ankle bone to 3 or 4 inches up the outer leg, this is usually due to excess supination. Worn out shoes, too many miles on a slanted road, or wearing shoes that have too much motion control for the individual are primary causes. Running on flat terrain, reducing mileage, and using a more neutral shoe can allow for healing.

- If the pain is sharp, and feels like it is on the bone, and none of the recommended treatments work, this could be a stress fracture. See a doctor.

- If the pain that developed gradually does not get better with rest and change of shoe, and the pain source seems to be in the region above or at the ankle bone, it could be a tear. This is especially true if it keeps reoccurring every time weekly mileage reaches a certain threshold. In this case there may or may not be mild swelling.

- If the ankle "goes out" as mentioned above, several weeks of no running may allow for healing, and the popping out (subluxation) may stop. But if subluxation has occurred a number of times, surgical repair may be needed.

- See a doctor if you suspect a tendon tear, stress fracture, or recurrent popping out of the tendons. There are several less common problems in this area as well.

- A doctor will usually need an MRI to determine if there is a tendon tear or to determine the cause of tendons popping out. An X-ray can often show a stress fracture in this area after 3 or 4 weeks. If a tendon is torn, it sometimes can heal without surgery, but normally this takes a long time. A period of immobilization can speed the healing if done soon after injury to get the healing started, but is usually not needed during the rest of the healing process. Many elect to have surgical repair because the results are usually good, but there is a risk of residual problems from any surgery. Subluxing, popping out tendons require surgery if the problem has been present for a long time. But if the feet are pronated or supinated, custom medical orthotics may correct the foot movement pattern of the ankle and take away the aggravation that leads to injury.

PEARLS

- All of the problems in this area have the potential to be managed and reduced over a very long period of time. It can take a couple of years for the internal ankle area to fully heal. Fragile tendons can continue to improve for a very long time if not aggravated. Many people have problems with popping out tendons in their teens but see gradual healing.

- Those with higher arched feet can experience post–ankle sprain pinching on the ankle bone due to pronation, even when they look straight when one is running in shoes. This type of foot has a limited ability to pronate at all, and even a small amount of over-normal pronation for the individual can be irritating. Finding a combination of shoes and inserts can bring the pronation into the "nonirritating" range for a temporary period.

WHEN TO STOP TRAINING

- The commonsense rules apply, but it is normal to train with a mild ache or soreness in this area—not pain.

CONSEQUENCES OF RUNNING OR WALKING THROUGH PAIN

- It is a mistake to continue training when there is pain or no progress in healing. Progression of the damage can occur just as well with long-term moderate pain as with short-term strong pain. Tendinitis will turn into a tear that requires surgery, and mild bone stress can become a stress fracture.

- It is unusual that pain starting in a single race would require a total training layoff. Staying below the threshold of irritation is the key. If the injury is not improving, a strategic healing period of 3 to 10 days can often jump start this process. Talk to your doctor.

INSIDE OF ANKLE—JUST ABOVE THE ANKLE BONE

TIBIALIS POSTERIOR ANKLE

LOCATION OF PAIN

- The tibialis posterior tendon and two others (flexor hallucis longus or flexor digitorum longus) will hurt on the inner ankle just above the ankle bone. The pain can be mistaken for bone pain.

- The pain is often located next to the tibia, at the ankle, or back toward the Achilles tendon and sometimes feels like Achilles tendinitis. Run your fingers up and down the Achilles tendon, and if there is pain, it is Achilles tendinitis. But if there is no pain, you may have medial tibia tendinitis. The affected tendons hide deeply behind the ankle bone, making it difficult to tell where the pain originates.

- If the bone hurts when you tap on it, you have a bone injury. Initial treatment is the same for MTT and bone injury in this region.

- This pain can be part of a broader injury that includes the muscles and tendons of the inner foot or inner leg.

DESCRIPTION OF PAIN

- Generally felt as an ache, pain can become a bit sharper as the foot lands on the ground.

- Soreness is possible when walking, but it should be mild. See a doctor if you experience strong pain.

- If there is sharp pain as the foot hits the ground, it may be a more extensive injury.

- Swelling is another sign of concern.

BASIC ANATOMY

- The tibialis posterior tendon extends from a muscle that attaches to the inner shin bone above the ankle. As it becomes a tendon, a few inches above the ankle bone, its job is to assist in foot propulsion. It also acts as a lever as it passes below the ankle bone to help the foot in a supination motion.

- The two tendons closer to the Achilles tendon can also become injured. It is important for a doctor to determine which is the problem, but the conservative treatment is the same, and the pain is similar.

- If the tendon is torn near the ankle bone, you have a serious problem.

- Stress fractures of the inner shin bone can occur just above the ankle bone. But a stress fracture on the prominent ankle bone itself is very serious and needs immediate attention. If the pain is felt on the back half of the prominent ankle bone, it is probably not this worrisome stress fracture, but if it is tender all the way toward the front of the bone, or if it is swollen, see a doctor.

CAUSES

- Excessive impact is usually a cause. Contributing factors can be shoes with poor cushioning, unaccustomed pavement running, long downhill runs, and adjustment to rigid orthotics.

- The most common cause is excessive pronation.

- Ankle sprains, even when the ankle rolls outward (inversion) may aggravate this area. This is not a common cause, but should be considered.

TREATMENT

- Standard icing (with ice bags or gel ice) and gentle massage is useful. This tendon and region can tolerate and improve with massage better than most tendons.

- Elimination of pronation while maintaining cushioning is important if you want to continue training. Some stability and motion control shoes have more cushioning than others. Neutral shoes are usually the most cushioned, but do not prevent pronation. A good combination may be a soft off-the-shelf orthotic in combination with a stable motion control shoe.

- Do not run if the pain does not disappear after a few minutes or if it returns during the run. A gentle soreness in the tendon is acceptable, not pain.

- An elastic ankle support may help. The kind designed for mild ankle sprains are usually comfortable and do not bother the ankle during training.

- If the pain does not improve or if it is very strong, a doctor should be consulted. The physical exam can determine if there is a tendon tear. It can also reveal the possibility of bone injury. X-rays are often negative but that does not mean that the bone is not damaged. Stress fractures are often difficult to see on an X-ray. Bone scans are more reliable, but do not reveal anything about the tendons. Most doctors would consider an MRI if anything beyond an X-ray was required. Physical therapy treatments are helpful unless the bone is injured, when rest is the best treatment. Ankle stress fractures heal at variable rates; 6 to 10 weeks is normal.

- Casts or crutches are not needed. If the stress fracture is on the prominent ankle bone itself, crutches are usually advised with a cast or removable cast boot. Allow a long time for healing. Sometimes it does not heal and surgery is needed. If it is determined that a tendon is torn, the extent of injury is important information. The further above the ankle bone, the more likely the tendon will heal without surgery. Sometimes there is no option but to repair the tendon with surgery.

PEARLS

- This pain can appear suddenly.

- The bone can be tender without being a stress fracture, similar to medial tibial stress syndrome in the leg pain section.

- Bone pain is more common when people are bow-legged.

- Tendon pain is more common in people who pronate excessively.

- Stretching provides little to no benefit in healing this injury.

- The tibialis posterior tendon is most commonly injured, and through the years it has become a broad term for pain in this area due to any cause.

WHEN TO STOP TRAINING

- Early rest is important to stop the damage in its earliest stage.

- Standard, common sense running/walking with pain, and returning to training rules apply.

CONSEQUENCES OF RUNNING OR WALKING THROUGH PAIN

- Mild stress to the bone can lead to serious stress fractures if pain is ignored.

- Mild tendinitis can become a tear with continued use.

- Pain in this area can appear suddenly during a race or training run. Sometimes this is the result of a sudden stress fracture, but this is unusual. In most cases it is tendinitis. Finishing the race in pain is an acceptable risk. If it is a stress fracture, it will require rest for several weeks afterward. If it is tendinitis, it may require rest if the pain remains. It is surprising how often athletes have pain during a race and a day or two later it is completely gone.

- Entering a race with a suspected stress fracture in this anatomical location is very risky. Nearly every experienced sports doctor has had a patient who developed a sudden complete fracture from this. These require surgery.

THROUGHOUT THE ANKLE—NO SPECIFIC AREA

RECURRENT INVERSION SPRAINS AND ANKLE INSTABILITY

LOCATION OF PAIN

- Pain may or may not be present as the ankle rolls easily and often beyond the normal range. This is commonly the reinjury of a serious inversion sprain, years earlier, that did not fully heal.

DESCRIPTION OF PAIN

- The instability of the ankle allows it to roll over easily—especially on uneven surfaces such as rugged trails. A more serious condition is noted when the ankle rolls over periodically on flat surfaces with no cause.

- When an ankle has rolled many times, there may be very little pain because the ligaments are so stretched they no longer become aggravated.

BASIC ANATOMY

- Those who stand or walk on the outer edges of their heels and feet are more likely to easily roll their ankles. Bowed legs can make this problem worse. Those who've had previous ankle sprains often have a more angled ankle with a reduced range of motion.

- During an inversion ankle sprain, the foot tilts inward under the leg bones. The top foot bone, the talus, fits inside a "pocket" made by the leg bones known as the tibia and fibula. The ankle ligaments hold the talus in this pocket. When the ligaments are stretched or torn, the talus tilts, allowing the outer edge to come out of the pocket. This also happens when the ligaments have been stretched permanently through recurrent sprains or from a serious sprain that never healed correctly. Pain occurs when the ligaments are injured. No pain occurs when the talus moves because the ligaments are permanently stretched out.

CAUSES

- Recurrent sprains are caused by structural weaknesses, previous injury, weak muscles, shoes with no lateral stability, the inability to adapt to uneven surfaces, running form irregularities, and performing other sports that involve contact or extreme lateral motion.

TREATMENT

- Conservative treatment begins with the proprioception balancing exercises (in the next section on ankle sprains).

- Three exercises can strengthen ankle support systems:

  1. Walk on the heels without letting the forefoot touch the ground for 1 minute.

  2. Walk on the outside of the feet without letting the big toe on each foot touch the ground for 1 minute.

  3. Walk on the inside of the feet without letting the little toe side of each foot touch the ground for 1 minute.

- These should be done while wearing shoes to avoid bruising the bones of the feet. They can be done every day for a while and then once or twice a week for maintenance.

- Some shoes help stabilize the footplant. Trail shoes generally have more lateral stability, and some models have cushioned midsoles that allow for road use. It's important that the shoe be the right width for your foot. Stand straight with the shoe tied. Look down at the outside of the shoe. A small portion of the midsole and sole should be visible along the full outer edge. If the upper overhangs the sole, it is easier for the shoe to roll over. Get a shoe with a wider base.

- Custom medical orthotics can help in stabilizing the outer edge of the foot to prevent sprains. It is almost impossible to find an off-the-shelf orthotic that provides good lateral stability.

- If an elastic ankle brace is worn constantly for running/walking, the ankle can become weaker and less stable when it is not worn. This can be prevented by doing the proprioception exercises and the strengthening exercises mentioned in the next section on ankle sprains. These exercises should be mandatory for those with unstable lateral ankle ligaments.

- When people begin training and racing on trails, they often have ankle instability. A gentle introduction to uneven terrain, while avoiding overuse, allows the leg and foot to adapt to this type of surface. Don't give up if this feels difficult.

- Running form changes can help decrease ankle sprains on uneven terrain. Most good trail runners have shorter strides with rapid stride frequency rates on rougher surfaces. Shorter strides are more stable.

- If the instability problems persist, consult a doctor, who can determine if the ligaments are permanently stretched or torn. This is important to know even if ankle rolling is infrequent. If the ligaments are torn, when the foot hits the ground, stopping the foot and talus, the ankle joint also stops. If the ligaments that stabilize the ankle are loose, the leg bone portion of the ankle joint can continue to move forward a few millimeters sliding on top of the talus. This friction can aggravate and damage the protective cartilage and eventually produce arthritis within the joint. This excess motion is reduced by strengthening/balance exercises, stable shoes, and ankle brace components. The intensity of workouts and racing can increase the damage. A doctor can determine if the range of motion in the ankle is too great or there are anatomical flaws that need extra support. If it is determined that the ligaments are not tight enough, surgery is a viable option and is usually successful.

PEARLS

- Even if it does not hurt, repeated episodes of ankle rolling produces damage that can lead to early arthritis.

- Both pronated feet and high arched feet can have unstable ankles. Reducing or eliminating the pronation will reduce instability. If a foot is heavily pronated at push-off, it will be supinating as it swings forward. Therefore, a misstep can push the foot into inversion and sprain. A normal foot will be neutral to slightly supinated at toe-off and will be pronating slightly as it strikes the ground. A misstep will not roll the foot outward.

- Surgically repaired ankles from fractures or ligament repair need the best stability available, which can be provided by medical orthotics. Often the ankle can change its position, angle, and flexibility. This means, in some cases, that different shoe models might be best for each foot, or at least a different orthotic angle for each.

WHEN TO STOP TRAINING

- Chronic pain or swelling without a recent sprain should be evaluated.

CONSEQUENCES OF RUNNING OR WALKING THROUGH PAIN

- Ankle arthritis is a strong possibility if recurrent sprains are ignored or if pain and swelling is persistent and no correction made.

TENDON JUST ABOVE THE BACK OF THE HEEL BONE

ACHILLES TENDON

LOCATION OF PAIN

- The pain can be anywhere along the tendon that attaches to the back of heel. It extends upward to the lower part of the calf muscle.

- Another area for pain is just above the heel, deeper than the tendon, but not near the ankle bones.

DESCRIPTION OF PAIN

- The mildest version does not hurt when exercising, but rather is a mild morning stiffness.

- It can progress to hurt for the first few minutes of a workout, and then go away.

- Some versions begin during a run, but are not felt afterward. Or it may hurt every few runs or walks. The frequency may increase gradually with pain felt the next morning.

- Running or walking up a hill will increase the pain, and going downhill may also aggravate it. The tendon bends when toes are lower than the heel and impact is greater going downhill. As the foot flattens and the ankle rolls, the Achilles tendon will twist.

- Sharp pain that begins suddenly during a run indicates a more severe injury.

- Swelling may or may not be present. This can be in the form of a bump on one side or cause the entire tendon to thicken, with soreness.

- Pain can vary from mild to severe.

BASIC ANATOMY

- The tendon originates at the lower portion of the calf. It is a broad strap at this point and actually blends into the calf muscle. It narrows as it travels downward toward the top of the heel bone and expands again as it attaches to the back of the heel.

- The narrow portion of the tendon is especially prone to injury because it has a poor blood supply and is compromised further when the tendon bends or twists.

- The tendon is enclosed in a type of sheath called the paratenon. This covering is as susceptible to injury and damage as the tendon.

- The tendon can be sore at the same time as the calf or the posterior heel bone because the same forces irritate all three.

CAUSES

- The tendon can handle the force of foot propulsion as long as 1) running mechanics are efficient, 2) there has been a gradual increase in intensity or distance, and 3) there has been sufficient rest between stresses to allow for adaptation. The tendon will become stronger and the connections will toughen as the stimulus of increased training triggers growth of tissue. Problems begin when improper motion irritates the tendon or the training workload is increased too quickly.

- Shoes that allow the heel to sit low, such as racing flats, can increase stress and trigger the pain. If you want to shift to a lower-heeled shoe, do so gradually.

- Pronation of the foot, especially among those with legs that are slightly bowed, can cause the tendon to bend and become C-shaped. This puts great stress on the tendon.

- The tendon can absorb the tremendous force of propulsion if the stress is distributed equally throughout. When the foot is pronated at push off, or is heavily pronated as it lands on the ground, the tendon becomes twisted. This overloads a portion of it because the force is uneven. This occurs anywhere along the tendon from the connection at the calf all the way down to the heel.

- Mild tendon soreness, the result of inflammation, is common when mileage is increased. There may be calf and heel soreness also. Ice massage every night (noted in Treatment) can reduce or eliminate the pain. If this low grade pain lasts for more than 10 days, seek treatment.

- A rapid tightening of the tendon usually combined with a twist can produce a tear or a rupture. Although the pain is sharp initially, a complete rupture may not hurt significantly. Sometimes the main complaint afterwards is loss of function in the forefoot and not being able to push off.

- A tendon that is injured is much more susceptible to rupture or tearing. This is extremely unlikely in normal running/walking. High risk activities include sprinting, hill running, and any motion that involves a sudden twist or unexpected tightening of the damaged tendon.

TREATMENT

- Icing with ice massage: Use a chunk of ice, and rub constantly on the tendon for 15 minutes. Ice bags and gel ice don't tend to provide a significant healing effect.

- Elevating the heel about a quarter of an inch with a lift in all shoes is surprisingly helpful.

- Stretching when the tendon has been recently injured should be avoided. As the tendon heals into its later stages, stretching can be added but is still a risk. It is best performed with the guidance of a doctor or therapist. Strengthening may be introduced at the same time. Normally tendons don't get stronger like muscles, but they can become adapted to higher loads through exercise.

- Focus on shoes and inserts first if there is a regular pattern of Achilles soreness. Overpronation or oversupination are often causes and can be controlled by more stable shoes and off-the-shelf orthotics. Once the tendon has been injury free for two months or more, it may be possible to move back to less stable shoes if one has used them successfully before the injury. After several tendon injuries occur, a stable shoe with medical orthotics can be helpful.

- Physical therapy, ultrasound, and other therapies are helpful. There is a special form of massage that can help with tendon pain and swelling, but it should not be overused for fear of irritating the tendon.

- Acupuncture can sometimes reduce the inflammation.

- Laser, electrical stimulation, and other modalities sometimes help.

- If the tendon is swollen, there is a bump on it, or you hear a noise when moving the ankle up and down, it must be rested.

- If the pain increases or persists more than a few weeks, see a doctor. Normally, X-rays do not show damage unless the pain is in the heel bone as well as the tendon. A good exam can lead to a diagnosis. If the doctor feels a defect or empty spot in the tendon, it is torn. Experienced doctors can determine whether the damage is to the paratenon (sheath) or to the tendon itself. The location of swelling or a bump can indicate how it was injured, and how difficult the healing process may be. Sometimes an MRI is necessary to see if there is permanent damage inside the tendon.

- When badly injured, a cast, or a cast boot can speed up the healing by immobilizing the foot.

- Never allow an injection into the tendon.

- In severe cases, surgery is sometimes necessary and the results are variable. Athletes have had success with surgical repair of ruptures, but this is debated. Tears do not need to be repaired unless they are fairly large, but a long break from sports is necessary to allow for healing. If the tendon itself is scarred and damaged internally, surgical repair can be effective. There is a chance, however, that the tendon will never be perfect again, but there may not be other options.

PEARLS

- Most athletes will have a few cases of sore Achilles tendons through the years. If intelligent care and a few rest days are taken at onset, training can be continued.

- High arches contribute to Achilles tendon problems and permanent use of heel lifts might be needed.

- Morning pain is often the last symptom to go away.

WHEN TO STOP TRAINING

- It is wise to rest two to four days when Achilles tendinitis first occurs. Use the ice massage and evaluate shoe choices.

- It is possible to start short workouts if the tendon feels normal after about two or three minutes into the workout. But if the pain returns during the workout, STOP.

- Continue training as long as the pain decreases.

CONSEQUENCES OF RUNNING OR WALKING THROUGH PAIN

- Tears and central tendon damage will occur if pain is ignored for weeks. Permanently temperamental tendons can be the result.

- Surgery may be required if the damage is extensive.

- It is possible to have gradual growth of strong pain during a difficult or extremely long race, without serious injury risk. Many runners who do this find that their tendons may be swollen and sore afterward. But if the pain gradually increased, it is extremely rare that permanent damage occurs. Runners who started the race with sore or injured tendons might cause permanent damage.

LOWER LEG BELOW THE KNEE

FRONT OF THE LOWER LEG—OUTSIDE OF THE SHIN BONE

ANTERIOR SHIN PAIN

LOCATION OF PAIN

- This shin pain is usually in the front of the leg. It can be along the front outer edge of the bone or more toward the inner leg, which is medial shin pain located on the shin bone, along the inner edge, or inside of the bone.

- Anterior shin pain is along the front crest of bone or just outside (lateral) in the muscle area next to the shin.

- Sometimes the front edge and the inner side are sore at the same time. Combining both treatments will help in this situation.

DESCRIPTION OF PAIN

- The pain can be mild and appear after workouts only. This is commonly associated with new athletes, rapid mileage changes, or an increase in the amount of speed training or racing. Running with an extended stride, especially on downhills or at the end of a strenuous run is often a cause.

- Slightly worse injury is indicated when it hurts at the beginning of a workout but goes away during the rest of the run, and then returns afterwards.

- Diffuse pain is safer than pain focused on a small spot. This is less worrisome than medial shin pain but requires attention and treatment.

- A more advanced injury is indicated if pain continues through the workout, especially if it hurts when walking, even if the pain is diffuse.

- A milder injury is present if there is no bone pain.

- Anterior pain is usually achy, as opposed to medial shin pain which may produce a burning sensation. Heel contact will often give the most intense pain, both in anterior and medial shin conditions. Medial shin pain will hurt more when the foot is flat and starts to push off.

- Impact is less of a cause, but the injury will feel somewhat better on softer surfaces.

- Hilly terrain will bother both conditions.

BASIC ANATOMY

- The group of muscles involved attach to the edge of the shin bone, just to the outside of the front edge. They extend from just above the ankle to about two to three inches below the knee. The tissue that connects them to the bone is a tough fibrous layer. When this tissue becomes stretched and damaged, the coating of the bone (periosteum) can become severely irritated and can progress to a stress reaction/stress fracture. The pulling of these muscles produces the pain. Anterior shin pain is much more likely to be due to injury or irritation of the muscle rather than the bone (as opposed to medial shin pain).

- The muscles lift the foot up at the ankle and let the foot down as the heel contacts the ground. The muscle strand closest to the bone also slows the pronation motion (rolling in) of the foot and ankle.

CAUSES

- Anterior shin pain is mostly a beginner's injury, but it may also occur due to a significant mileage increase or running too much on unstable terrain. Each foot is raised and lowered more than 700 times every mile. Gentle increases in training will naturally condition the lifting muscles in the front of the shin, but too much of an increase will overwhelm them.

- Tight calf muscles can put more workload on the lifting muscles in the front.

- Excessive pronation can overwhelm the small muscles that try to control this motion at heel contact.

- All of these motions are exaggerated on hills or when running faster.

- An exaggerated heel strike with the toes high in the air is also a cause.

- In a minority of shin pain cases in this area, exercise-induced chronic compartment syndrome could be present. This is produced when the shin muscles experience a rapid expansion but are contained by the sheath of connective tissue surrounding it, which is tough and inelastic. The sudden increase in pressure causes significant pain and sometimes loss of function due to a reduction of the blood supply. The blood does not flow normally when the pressure in the compartment is too high. See a doctor if there is a consistent threshold when the pain begins, numbness or tingling before or during the pain, and loss of normal function of the foot ankle. Compartment syndrome symptoms are relieved almost immediately by stopping, and one is able to return to activity without symptoms after a short rest. General progression is indicated with a return of the symptoms during progressively shorter intervals of running. Sometimes the foot will feel like it slaps and stops working during normal anterior shin pain also. In this case, normal fatigue/nerve irritation can be the cause. Because compartment syndrome is rare, seeing a doctor is not advised unless it persists. A longer and more gentle warm-up can help in some cases. When pace is reduced and more walk breaks are used, the legs often adapt and the problem goes away.

TREATMENT

- Icing and massage initially.

- Decrease mileage. Sometimes approximately five days off from running are needed, but not as often as when experiencing medial shin pain.

- If it is clear that the calves are tight, careful stretching and massage done gently can help.

- Excessive pronation is related to anterior conditions, but this is more commonly a cause of medial shin pain. Get a shoe check from experienced shoe experts and replace shoes if the midsole is not supporting as needed, or if another model could support better.

- This pain is much more likely to go away with conservative treatment while continuing to run when staying below the threshold of irritation.

- Evaluate running stride for excessive heel contact.

- If mild compartment syndrome symptoms are suspected, be very aggressive with the massage, make sure your shoes are cushioned adequately, and reduce the supination (rolling out) of the foot. Gentle stretching of the calves helps in some cases. Ease back into training below the level of pain.

- If the pain is caused by running, frequent walk breaks can allow for recovery and often will permit longer workouts.

- Early in the season or when first beginning to train, it is helpful to walk on the backs of the heels without letting the toes touch the ground for a minute before each workout to strengthen the anterior shin muscles. It is risky to do too much strengthening when they are very sore, however.

- If the pain is intense or will not go away with rest, see a doctor. X-rays may reveal a stress fracture if the pain is on the bone. X-rays of stress fractures are easier to see on the anterior bone than when medial shin stress fractures are present, but both may not show on an X-ray. Bone scans or MRIs are more revealing. Extended rest is the treatment for this condition.

- If a compartment syndrome injury is suspected, a pressure measurement test can be performed. This requires placing a needle with a gauge into the compartment when the shin is hurting. Unlike the medial compartment, surgery to expand the anterior compartment is quite effective and works within a few weeks, but fortunately is not always required. It is common for the compartment problem to gradually go away through a reduction in duration and intensity of training, more rest days, a better warm-up, and massage. But sometimes, time off from running is needed (9 to 12 months).

- Physical therapy can be quite effective in speeding up the healing process except for stress fractures.

PEARLS

- A high percentage of beginners have anterior shin pain.

- Most can train through this injury.

- High arches, tight calves, high body mass, and too much supination can predispose people to this injury.

WHEN TO STOP TRAINING

- If the pain becomes sharply focused, if the foot loses function more than once or twice, or if each workout is causing a rapid increase in symptoms, stop training.

CONSEQUENCES OF RUNNING OR WALKING THROUGH PAIN

- In most cases, anterior shin pain allows for continued training, under the guidelines listed.

FRONT OF THE SHIN—ON THE INSIDE INNER EDGE

MEDIAL SHIN PAIN

LOCATION OF PAIN

- Medial shin pain is usually in the front of the shin more toward the inner edge, or deep inside the bone.

- Sometimes the front edge (anterior shin pain) and the inner side are sore at the same time. Combining treatments for both usually helps.

DESCRIPTION OF PAIN

- The pain can be mild and appear after workouts only. This is commonly associated with new exercisers or a rapid mileage or intensity increase.

- A slightly worse injury is indicated when there is pain at the beginning of a workout, which goes away during exercise and returns afterward.

- Diffuse pain usually denotes a less serious injury than pain from a small spot.

- Pain that continues through the workout and especially when walking indicates a more advanced injury even if the pain is diffuse.

- Pain that involves the bone is a more serious injury.

BASIC ANATOMY

- The group of muscles involved are attached to the edge of the shin bone, just to the inside of the front edge. They extend from just above the ankle to about two to three inches below the knee. The tissue that connects them to the bone is a tough fibrous layer. When this tissue becomes stretched and damaged, the coating of the bone (periosteum) can become severely irritated and can progress to a stress reaction/stress fracture. The pulling of these muscles produces the pain. Anterior shin pain is much more likely to be due to injury/irritation of the muscle rather than the bone (as opposed to medial shin pain).

- The bone can be inflamed by impact. The resulting bone pain is usually diffuse and achy. The bone will eventually adapt, becoming more sturdy and dense, resulting in a reduction or cessation of the original soreness. But if the bone does not adapt, damage may progress into a stress fracture. These fractures are often transverse, running across the bone.

- Shin pain from the bone is due to impact and leg motion, and may occur in a variety of locations. Depending upon the problem, the treatment may be focused on impact or on motion control.

- Medial shin pain can also be located in the muscles and tendons when they absorb the force of the foot striking the ground. The cause is usually from excess motion and lack of conditioning.

- "Shin splints" is a general term for any pain in the leg near the front or inner side of the lower leg caused by running or walking. Pain along the inner portion, as described, is sometimes called medial tibial stress syndrome or MTSS. Using the term medial shin splints can differentiate it from pain in the front (anterior shin pain). Pain that is in the soft tissue on the inside of the lower leg is called posterior tibialis myositis or tendinitis. If in the middle or upper leg, soft tissue pain is called medial soleus myositis or tendinitis.

- In a minority of shin pain cases in this area, exercise-induced chronic compartment syndrome could be present. This is produced when the shin muscles experience a rapid expansion but are contained by the tough and inelastic sheath of connective tissue surrounding it. The sudden increase in pressure causes significant pain and sometimes loss of function due to a reduction of the blood supply. The blood does not flow normally when the pressure in the compartment is too high. See a doctor if there is a consistent threshold when the pain begins, there is numbness or tingling before or during the pain, and loss of normal function of the foot or ankle. Compartment syndrome symptoms are relieved almost immediately by stopping, and one is able to return to activity without symptoms after a short rest. General progression is indicated with a return of the symptoms during progressively shorter intervals of running. Sometimes the foot will feel like it slaps and stops working during normal posterior shin pain also. In this case, normal fatigue or nerve irritation can be the cause. Because compartment syndrome is rare, seeing a doctor is not advised unless it persists. A longer and more gentle warm-up can help in some cases. When pace is reduced and more walk breaks are used, the legs often adapt and the problem goes away.

CAUSES

- Pain is caused by the muscles or bone taking on more stress than they are used to absorbing. For some, this occurs at very low distance. Veterans may experience this injury due to progressive stress, lack of strategic rest, or both.

- Excessive pronation (rolling in) is a major cause of medial shin pain.

- Athletes with bowed legs are more likely to have problems because of the tendency of the bone to flex more at impact and because the foot is pronated more relative to the leg (it angles at the ankle). This may be the case even if the shoe is straight relative to the ground.

- Excessive impact can be due to inadequate shoe cushion, running on hard surfaces, running form irregularities, downhill running, large body mass, rigid higher arched feet, faster running, and mileage or intensity increases.

TREATMENT

- Treat the painful area initially with ice and massage. The massage may hurt, so icing prior to massage will help.

- Reduce mileage and add rest days, if needed.

- Run on softer surfaces. Avoid hills. Warm up gradually. Don't do any fast running.

- Get a shoe check in a technical running store. Shoes in the "stability" or "motion control" categories are suggested. When a shoe has a stable platform, excess pronation can be reduced or managed. Stability is much more important than cushion. Softer shoes are usually less stable. If you feel the need for more cushioning, use soft insoles or gel heel cups.

- Shin compression sleeves, support socks, or shin taping can often help in milder cases.

- Staying below the threshold of further irritation can allow most to run while the injury heals, and can help the shins adapt and become stronger (not in severe cases).

- It is common to experience shin pain when starting to run again after a layoff of several weeks or months. Athletes who are fit from other sports (such as cyclists) are particularly vulnerable. They have the fitness to go farther than the shins can handle. Minimal running during the "off" season (even one running day a week) can reduce the chance of shin pain. It's okay to run on treadmills for this minimal maintenance.

- See a doctor if the pain persists despite these measures.

- Stress fractures are usually indicated by an increase in pain as one continues to run. In most cases, extended rest is needed and will usually allow for complete healing. Linear stress fractures that developed gradually and became intense over time can require months to heal. Sudden stress fractures heal more quickly in about 8 to 10 weeks. Soft tissue shin pain and mild bone pain can heal in two to six weeks.

- Stress fracture diagnosis: A doctor would examine the shin, looking for a bump on the bone, thickening of the connective tissue, and any specific area that is sensitive. The way the foot functions and the quantity of pronation should also be determined—usually by a running gait analysis. An X-ray may be suggested, but a majority of stress fractures never show. A bone scan or MRI is more accurate. Primary treatment for stress fractures is rest. Casts are usually not required. Many doctors make the diagnosis through exclusion. If the pain is intense and does not respond to available treatment, it is probably a stress fracture.

- Physical therapy can help speed the healing. This can include many modalities. Stretching for medial shin pain is not very helpful, but strengthening can help.

- If there is pain when walking, a walking cast boot (or boot cast) can speed the healing. Sometimes this only needs to be worn when active and can be removed at home or when sleeping.

- Injections in the shin can help, but this is only useful for specific types of shin pain.

- Custom medical orthotics are valuable for longer term injuries, recurrent injuries, or for pronators who need to wear lighter shoes (such as racing or hard trail running shoes which do not provide as much anti-pronation design).

- Temporary or off-the-shelf orthotics, especially if provided by a knowledgeable doctor, can be very effective.

PEARLS

- Some runners are more prone to shin pain due to their anatomy. This is nearly always curable with very gradual mileage increases, strategic rest, more frequent walk breaks, careful shoe choices, orthotics, and possibly strengthening.

- Softer orthotics may provide relief when the shins are sore, but firmer ones can protect from reinjury.

- Many orthotics fail to cure the problem. It is important to choose a doctor who is very experienced in the fabrication and design of orthotics to increase the success rate of the treatment.

- Running gait analysis will provide valuable information for treatment.

- Icing and massage, even if painful, can be very helpful.

- Stress fractures that begin gradually and evolve over time produce a lot of soft tissue damage also. Following the treatment plan for non-stress fracture shin pain, with rest, will shorten the time needed to return to training after the bone heals.

- Sudden onset stress fractures do not require therapy because the problem is almost totally confined to the bone—unless this is caused by weak muscles or structural weakness.

WHEN TO STOP TRAINING

- Continued training is usually fine if there is mild to moderate shin pain that goes away during the first five minutes of a workout, is not felt during the rest of the workout, does not hurt with daily walking (even if it is sore after a run). If the pain does not recover to its previous level by the next day, more rest is needed.

- If it hurts with daily activity, do not train.

- If pain returns during a workout, STOP.

- Increasing walk breaks may allow one to run while the shin injury is healing (not with stress fractures).

CONSEQUENCES OF RUNNING OR WALKING THROUGH PAIN

- If the pain remains through a workout, it can progress to a more serious injury.

- Muscular pain can become bone pain which can result in a stress fracture and in rare cases a true fracture requiring surgery.

- A single episode of pain that appears late in a race might turn out to be a mild muscle injury. It might also be more extensive and require prolonged rest to heal. If the race is important and the rest is acceptable, the risk of permanent or extremely long-term injury is low.

OUTSIDE OF THE LOWER LEG—ABOVE THE ANKLE TO JUST BELOW THE KNEE

LATERAL LOWER LEG PAIN

LOCATION OF PAIN

- Pain is experienced along the outer leg from a couple of inches above the ankle bone to a couple of inches below the knee, it can be directly on top of the outer leg bone (fibula), in front of it, or just behind.

DESCRIPTION OF PAIN

- This is usually an achy, diffuse pain. On rare occasions it is deep, sharp, and focused in a small area.

- During a workout it is common to experience a pain increase with lingering pain afterward during daily activity. Rest usually settles it down.

- Often, there is pain only during the first part of a workout.

- The sharper, deep pain usually comes directly from the bone, hurts when pressured, and is usually the result of continuing to train when previously sore. On rare occasions it can appear suddenly.

- After an ankle sprain there can be soreness in this area.

BASIC ANATOMY

- The lateral muscles lift the outside of the foot and prevent excess supination. They attach to the outer leg bone (fibula).

- These muscles are also used when running at a fast pace, especially when sprinting.

- The fibula can suffer a stress fracture.

CAUSES

- Excess supination is a primary cause of pain in this area.

- General muscle soreness is usually indicated by diffuse achy pain, in both legs, after or during a faster run or race. The soreness is not necessarily due to excess supination.

- Ankle sprains can stretch and injure these muscles and the associated tendons and ligaments.

- The fibula bone absorbs a significant amount of twisting or torque while running. Impact from faster running, and the resulting strong pull of the muscles, will increase pressure on the bone producing a stress fracture if the bone cannot adapt. These are not common.

TREATMENT

- Ice and massage are effective initial treatments.

- Mild overpronation can reduce stress on the lateral muscles and allow for continued training during the healing process.

- Shoes with at least some stability can speed up healing. Experienced staff at a technical running store can help you find a good match for your foot. When experiencing recurring or slow healing injuries, some runners can use shoes that are not as rigid.

- Sharp strong pain, especially if localized, should be checked by a doctor. Strong pain, caused by an ankle issue, should also be checked by a medical specialist. An inversion sprain can sometimes lead to a fracture higher up the leg, on the outside.

- An X-ray can usually determine if a stress fracture is present, but sometimes a bone scan or MRI is needed. Physical therapy is also helpful in many non fracture cases.

PEARLS

- When the injury is treated early, continued training is almost always possible, if the runner/walker stays below the threshold of irritation.

- This muscle group can cramp from overuse, caused by too much exercise, too soon, and dehydration or electrolyte imbalance. More frequent walk breaks can usually eliminate the cramping.

WHEN TO STOP TRAINING

- Sharp strong pain can indicate the early stages of a stress fracture. Take time off from training and see a doctor.

- Swelling and pain during daily walking indicates a more serious injury that requires rest and diagnosis.

CONSEQUENCES OF RUNNING OR WALKING THROUGH PAIN

- Pain that gradually begins during a race or workout is common and usually can allow for continued training. If the pain is strong, use common sense and stop if necessary.

- Continuing to train regularly with strong pain is risky because muscle injury can progress and eventually evolve into a much more long-term injury, such as a stress fracture.

NOTE: Since you lose no conditioning by resting for as long as five days, it is always better to take extra days off if you suspect a serious problem.

VARIOUS PAINS IN THE CALF MUSCLE

CALF PAIN

LOCATION OF PAIN

- The calf is a large, fleshy group of muscles on the backside of the lower leg between the knee and the Achilles tendon. Pain on the inner side is called "medial" while "lateral" refers to the outside and back of the calf.

- Pain may be felt throughout the calf muscle, or in a specific place. Since the Achilles connects directly into the calf muscle, pain may be noticed in that tendon. If this is the case, look at the Achilles Tendinitis section in this book.

- A single episode of calf soreness is of no concern if there is a reason and it goes away.

DESCRIPTION OF PAIN

- The pain is often a mild general ache that appears after a run in both calf muscles. This is usually minor training soreness if associated with a change in distance, effort, shoes, or an increase in hilly terrain. It is also common for one calf to be more sore than the other.

- Another type of pain may occur during a run, usually to one calf. Sometimes pain gradually increases but can also be sharp and sudden. The calf may remain sore after the run when walking. Sometimes the pain appears unexpectedly after it seemed to have gone away. This can be during the next run or several runs later. Many runners are susceptible to frequent episodes several times a year. There may or may not be swelling in the muscle, a thickened spot, a "knot" or a defect.

- Cramping is the sudden contraction of the calf muscle which can restrict or prohibit use of the muscle. This may occur at night or during a run, and usually goes away with rest. Cramping may become chronic and last for weeks when training is suddenly increased, or continuously increased over days or weeks without adequate rest. Inadequate use of walk breaks from the beginning of a run is another common cause.

BASIC ANATOMY

- The two primary muscles in the calf are the gastrocnemius and soleus. The soleus is the deeper muscle farther down the leg, and the gastrocnemius is higher and on the outside.

- These muscles attach to the back of the leg bone and flow into and become the Achilles tendon. They provide most of the power for running.

- There is a significant amount of connective tissue interspersed throughout the muscles that can get injured with or without the muscle mass being damaged.

- Generalized soreness from training is caused by mild connective tissue damage. When muscle cells are pushed beyond their current capacity, they can be damaged. With sufficient rest, the muscles will be strengthened as they adapt to more efficient running. But when muscle cells are repeatedly abused, more and more areas break down and a strain or tear may occur.

- The most common calf injury is called a strain. This is often due to strong strands of muscle fiber continually pulling so hard that they tear the tiny connections to uninjured muscle fibers nearby. This injury usually occurs suddenly during a run. There might be a thickened area near the pain. At first there is often some swelling. After a few days, firm connective tissue forms at the site. Some call these "knots" and can be felt during a deep tissue massage.

- A calf muscle tear is the result of damage to the muscle cells and connective tissue. This is a more serious injury.

- Calf cramping is caused by uncontrollable firing of the muscle or portion of the muscle due to overuse or dehydration. This can be significantly aggravated by an imbalance of the chemicals in and around the muscle cells during hard or prolonged exercise. A less common reason for cramping is poor circulation during exercise or when at rest, often producing a deep ache. Inadequate frequency of walk breaks is often a cause of cramping.

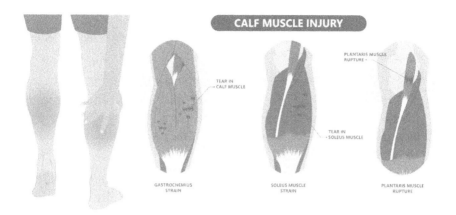

CALF MUSCLE INJURY

GASTROCNEMIUS STRAIN

TEAR IN CALF MUSCLE

SOLEUS MUSCLE STRAIN

TEAR IN SOLEUS MUSCLE

PLANTARIS MUSCLE RUPTURE

PLANTARIS MUSCLE RUPTURE

CAUSES

- Strains and tears can occur because of a single excessive effort, even as little as missing a step.

- **NOTE:** Jeff has worked with a number of runners who suffered from strains or tears by stretching routines, especially when the muscle was fatigued from exercise.

- A strain or tear that occurs for no apparent reason is mostly commonly due to lack of strength, but sometimes due to lack of flexibility.

- Excessive pronation and supination will overload a portion of the muscle because the force is not being distributed evenly as the foot straightens out, especially if the injury is toward the outer or inner portion of the muscle.

- Cramping can be caused by fatigue due to continuous use, and dehydration/ loss of electrolytes during a strenuous or prolonged workout or race.

- Cramping that occurs without a known reason may be related to decreasing circulation. This is called claudication and should be checked by a doctor.

TREATMENT

- Normal muscle soreness will recover with rest, ice, and massage. It is not necessary for the soreness to be completely gone to resume training. Shorter workouts, slower pacing from the beginning and more frequent walk breaks will often allow for training while the soreness abates. If the pain increases during a workout, even after taking a rest interval and reducing the effort significantly, stop.

- Massage has been very effective in treating calf muscle problems. See an experienced sports massage therapist who has successfully treated runners with the type of problems you are having. Be gentle with massage immediately after the injury occurred. Read the next section on calf tears/ massage.

- Stretching is risky and can damage a tear or strain further, and often aggravates a calf muscle cramp. Don't push the muscle into a stretch if you feel pain or damage.

- A strain should be treated with ice and very gentle massage initially. Heel pads, heel lifts, or moderately elevated shoes should be worn. Avoid stretching until healing is well underway, if then. Strains do not require a cast or walking boot unless they are very painful. After a few days, the intensity of the massage can increase. Most mild strains become almost painless during everyday activity after about two weeks. At this point an exercise, such as calf raises, should be added. While standing on a floor (these should not be done on an incline – the heel, should be on the same surface as the forefoot) rise up onto the forefoot lifting the heels up as high as possible standing on tiptoe. Lower slowly to the ground. Do this 25 times if possible without pain or fatigue. Stop if the injury begins to hurt. When able to do 25, modify the exercise where 25 are done with the toes pointing toward each other (pigeon-toed). Then immediately do 25 with the toes pointing out (duck-footed). This raises the total to 50 overall. When this can be done without causing the injury to hurt, it is okay to begin trying to return to training. It may take days to a couple of weeks to achieve the goal. If this is not done, reinjury is quite common.

- Calf tears may require immobilization if they are severe. If there is significant calf pain and a tear is suspected, see a doctor. A cast or walking boot can allow the defect in the muscle to heal. Treatment for mild tears, or tears that are almost healed, can be the same as that for strains except that massage should be delayed until later stages. It is important for the repaired tissue to bridge the tear before using massage. Tears normally take much longer than strains to heal.

- See a doctor if the pain is strong, if there is a depression in the muscle, if swelling and redness is obvious, or if cramping is from an unknown source. It is common for a doctor to recommend physical therapy, which can speed up the healing process.

- Reoccurring calf injuries indicate muscle damage or defective muscle tissue. These may occur as training is resumed or randomly, every few months. Lack of flexibility is overemphasized as a cause of this problem. There is no doubt that tight calves contribute to greater load on the calf, but many people with extremely tight calves never get injured. Strength is the overlooked variable. Strong calves are more difficult to injure and weak calves can be injured more easily. Just because a calf is large does not mean it has adequate strength to resist injury. When people run or walk, they need to push off for propulsion. The push is provided mostly by the calf muscle cells firing causing the muscle to contract. As connective tissue in the calf contracts and stretches during the running motion, it rebounds like a spring providing power to the ankle, adding to the mechanical action of the ankle. When calves are excessively tight, the muscles work less because the connective tissue is stretched further and does more of the propulsion. A subtle weakening of the muscles itself can occur. Any demand beyond the strength of the connective tissue will cause it to tear. The muscle needs to be strong to help the connective tissue and protect it.

This kind of strength is very specific. Standard weight training is not as effective as exercise done in the running motion (hills, longer and slower workouts). After the injury has recovered by using the previously mentioned treatments, including calf raises, and training is beginning, it is necessary to gradually overload the calves in a controlled manner. Coaches do this with runners by gradually adding specific workouts. A series of hill repeat workouts, for example, can precede track workouts and longer distance track repeats are scheduled before moving to shorter, more intense distances. Average runners or walkers can improve strength by performing 15 or 20 minutes of "springy striding" once or twice a week. This is nothing more than running or walking with a little more bouncy stride than necessary, after a 10 minute warm-up of gentle running. This is not jumping or bounding. If done correctly, only you will know when you are doing it. An observer might notice that you have a nice lively stride. We often do this anyway when we feel really energetic or at the end of a short workout. These exercises should be done in the middle of an easy day, not during a long or hard workout. Maintaining this routine is especially important for anyone who has had a problem with their calves and especially those who tend to run the same distance each day, maintaining the same weekly mileage. If the exercise is neglected, after a period of time, the calf injury pattern can return.

- The common causes of calf injuries are the following: unequal leg length, excessive pronation and supination, extremely tight calves, rigid high arches, and large body mass. Leg length differences are best determined by a medical professional, but the clues are the following: unequal shoe wear, pant leg length differences, and an obvious difference when standing in front of a mirror. The calf injury can occur on either the long or short side—but usually on the short side. Pronation and supination can be managed with shoe changes and orthotics. The effect of tight calves can be reversed by choosing shoes that are not low in the heels and by using thin heel lifts. Many people use lifts throughout their running/walking careers. Those with rigid high arches can receive relief with heel padding as a gentle lift. Getting good shoe advice can help greatly. High body mass stresses the calves, and may require treatment even when fewer signs of structural flaws are present. More frequent walk breaks from the beginning of runs has reduced calf problems—especially for heavier runners.

PEARLS

- Recurrent calf injuries are common as athletes grow older, often due to the reduction in daily physical activity. Alternate exercise and sports are forgotten and weakness gradually sets in. Recovery time increases with increasing age, and tissue damage heals more slowly.

- Working out on soft surfaces where the heel sinks down is sometimes a cause (in sand or snow).

- Jump rope and calf raises with additional weight can injure the calf muscle unexpectedly.

WHEN TO STOP TRAINING

- If the pain increases during workouts, there is noticeable pain with daily activity, or if the calf is more sore after a test workout, STOP!

CONSEQUENCES OF RUNNING OR WALKING THROUGH PAIN

- If ignored, a sore muscle can become a strain and then a tear. Either of these will require an extended recovery period. It is unusual that a serious condition would occur during a single run. So it is logical to consider finishing an important race when there is minor or average soreness. If calf pain occurs during a run, walk for several minutes. If it is a cramp, stop and massage the area, then walk for a few minutes and ease back into your pace. Remember to practice good hydration with adequate ingestion of fluids and electrolytes.

THE KNEE

PAIN AT THE KNEECAP OR AT THE MUSCLE ATTACHMENT AT THE KNEECAP

PATELLO-FEMORAL KNEE PAIN

LOCATION OF PAIN

- This injury can be located in the area from the top of the kneecap down to the bump on the top of the leg bone, just below the kneecap (tibial tuberosity or tibial tubercle), stretching an inch on either side of the kneecap.

DESCRIPTION OF PAIN

- When there is pain at the muscle attachment on the top of the kneecap, treat it immediately. If this area gets irritated, it can be persistent and respond slowly to rest. This condition rarely becomes intense, but can cause a major interruption in training. If this type of pain is due to a fall, the muscle can become detached, is quite painful, and often swollen.

- Pain at the kneecap can be variable. It may feel only slightly achy to very painful, forcing one to limp. Sensations may seem to come from the surface of the kneecap or from deep inside, and often produce sounds, such as clicking, crunching, popping, and catching. Sometimes the pain is along either or both edges. When this area is seriously injured, there will be swelling throughout the knee.

- Pain at the bottom of the kneecap. If deep, it is related to the kneecap problems mentioned previously. But lower knee pain, near the surface, is often a variation of tendinitis of the patellar tendon, which connects the kneecap to the front of the leg bone. Pain may also be experienced in the tendon itself and on the prominent bony connection point at the front of the upper leg bone (tibial tuberosity or tibial tubercle). When this tendon connection point is injured, it usually hurts when kneeling. The irritated area can grow in size when sore and may remain permanently enlarged and painful (especially in young people). Running downhill is stressful and painful for all tendon injuries. The pain can be very persistent and may vary from a constant soreness to periods of strong pain mixed with little pain. Sometimes the tendon can swell and be painful when squeezed.

- Pain along the edges of the kneecap is typically mild to moderate and usually improves with rest. More serious problems are possible when the pain is deeper near the edges, particularly when it is at the joint line of the knee.

BASIC ANATOMY

- The knee is a hinge joint as it hinges, the kneecap slides in a groove along the front. The powerful thigh muscles transition into the patellar tendon at the bottom of the kneecap. This important tendon extends a couple of inches to the top of the leg bone, where it attaches at the tibial tuberosity – a bump on the bone in the front. Where there is friction you'll find a layer of protective cartilage. The irritation and damaging of the cartilage produces a form of arthritis.

- The meniscus is another tissue in the knee that can become injured. This is a wedge shaped like a half moon that fits between the thigh bone (femur) and the leg bone (tibia). There are two of them in each knee. They provide cushion and hold the bones in perfect position minimizing friction when the knee hinges. They are composed of a type of cartilage called fibrocartilage. When the knee is twisted into an unstable and inefficient position, or if one of the bones moves excessively, the meniscus can be pinched or torn, which is painful. Damaged meniscus may cause the normal cartilage near the meniscus to gradually wear down.

CAUSES

- The top of the kneecap is commonly injured when there is too much pulling stress at the thigh muscle connection. This is an area that can adapt to increasing load. But too much downhill running, mileage increases, sudden unexpected stress from weight training (especially when lifting too much weight), jumping, landing in the wrong position, etc. are all causes.

- Pain at the kneecap itself is also load-related. If the cartilage between the kneecap and femur is not adequately adapted, it can become irritated. The cartilage will become thicker and stronger if the adaptation is gradual. There is a wide variability among individuals as to the amount of time needed. If the irritation continues, it can result in arthritis of the cartilage surface and be permanently susceptible to pain. If the surfaces do not match closely, if the knee is inflamed and the fluid inside the knee is changed from normal because of inflammation, or if the cartilage surface is damaged, you may hear clicking, popping, or crunching. Sometimes this goes away as the knee heals, but if it persists, or is new and significant, see a doctor. Some people experience this from a young age and accept it as normal. Many people have shallow patellar grooves at the back of the kneecap, or an irregularly shaped knee cap which can produce more friction as the knee cap slides. If a person has bowed legs or knock knees, the kneecap can also slide a bit sideways when the knee bends, which exerts more pressure on the area. Excessive foot pronation or supination causes the knee to turn in or out and stresses the knee.

- Pain along the lateral edges of the kneecap is usually an irritation of the connective tissue that holds the kneecap aligned in its groove. When the forces applied to the kneecap pull it sideways, the connective tissue becomes irritated. Anatomical variations mentioned earlier are causes, but excessive pronation and supination are also often causes.

- Pain in the patellar tendon is related to excessive load, so gradual adaptation will help. The individual anatomical shape of the knee affects the direction of pull at the patellar tendon. Pulling at an angle results in more stress to the tendon. Excessive pronation and sometimes supination is related and often overlooked as a cause. If the tendon is significantly injured or pain is ignored for a long period of time, the tendon can become permanently damaged.

- Pain at the tendon insertion, on the tibial tuberosity, is caused by the same factors that produce patellar tendon pain. Pronation and supination are less of a cause, though. Young people, especially boys up to about 16 years old, have a growth center in this area that can become irritated.

TREATMENT

- Mild knee pain is normal as long as there is a logical reason for it. Increased mileage, shoe changes, hills, or other sports or exercises are typical causes. It is fine to train through mild pain because the knee will gradually adapt. If the pain does not follow commonsense "running with pain rules," rest is very important.

- See a doctor if there is swelling, or if the pain is sharp, strong, or recurrent. Long- term, low grade pain that is ignored is a common indication of internal irritation that can result in irreversible knee damage.

- Typical pain around the patella, other than the patellar tendon, is treated in several ways. Always evaluate the shoes for stability. Custom medical orthotics may be required for people with anatomical variability so that the knee is aligned. This is very effective for recurrent mild pain especially when the sensation appears fairly consistently at a certain threshold.

- Thigh muscle (quadriceps) strength is very important in holding the patella in alignment and in decreasing excessive knee movement. The inner muscle called the vastus medialis oblique (VMO) is where the focus should be applied. VMO exercises take time to provide value, but can protect the knee from future injuries. While muscles get stronger through adaptation, some runners need to work a lot more than others to realize the benefits, with rest between workouts.

- Patellar tendon and tibial tuberosity pain indicates a need for rest—if the pain is not reduced significantly due to a commonsense running plan reduction. These areas heal very slowly if they are strongly irritated. Massage to the tendon and ice massage may help. Patellar tendon straps may allow for continued training.

- Elastic knee sleeves, patellar tendon straps, and knee braces may be useful for any knee pain. Results vary widely among products and among individuals. So if one sleeve has not helped, another one may.

- Physical therapists and trainers use a patellar taping method that is useful.

PEARLS

- Running does not cause damage to knees unless it is done when there is pain or swelling. Studies have shown thicker cartilage and healthier knees even in high mileage runners due to adaptation.

- Many runners get arthritis because they have a genetic tendency to have arthritis and would get it whether they run or not. There is a wide variability from person to person in susceptibility.

- Many people who have to stop continuous running because of arthritis can sometimes run when using liberal walk breaks. Others who have arthritic pain when running have no pain when walking and doing everyday activities. Many average, nonrunning citizens have unknown arthritis and don't do enough activity to discover the symptoms.

- Surgery should be considered very carefully because knees are never the same after surgery. Some tissue is nearly always removed which will put more stress on the remaining surfaces. Anterior cruciate ligament repair often provides good results for running/walking, but patellar cartilage debridement (shaving) has a poor outcome. Lateral releases (to cut the tissue that holds the kneecap to the outside) are overused but can be helpful in the rare situations where it is truly the cause of the pain. Through the years, trends in knee surgery, like lateral release, have come and gone. Years ago surgery on plica (a band of connective tissue found in many knees) was routinely performed. It is much less common now. Orthopedists have become more conservative and tend to leave more of the meniscus (rather than aggressively "cleaning it up"). Promising new procedures can provide surfaces to eliminate "bone on bone" friction from cartilage-deficient areas. Nonsurgical, injectable hyaluronic acid provides surface area and lubrication. All of these options should be discussed with your orthopedist, and second opinions should be considered.

WHEN TO STOP TRAINING

- Most athletes will have knee pain periodically. As the knees adapt to increasing stress, a normal amount of irritation will occur. If it is mild, goes away after warm-up or during training, and continues to improve, it is generally safe to work out. When pain is in both knees, it is usually an adaptation issue. Running every other day and including liberal walk breaks can reduce or eliminate the problem in many cases. Knee injuries are the most common reason why athletes to have to permanently change their activity or retire from an activity. Rest and treatment should be started immediately if the pain persists.

CONSEQUENCES OF RUNNING OR WALKING THROUGH PAIN

- Knee pain is often mild to moderate, so it is easy to ignore it for long periods of time. But permanent damage can occur gradually without strong pain ever being present. Be conservative!

THE AREA DIRECTLY BEHIND AND TOWARD THE INSIDE OF THE KNEE

POPLITEAL AND PES ANSERINUS PAIN

LOCATION OF PAIN

- Popliteal pain is felt directly in the back of the knee, toward the inside or middle of the back of the knee. The outer border is the biceps femoris tendon (toward the outside at the back of the knee) and is discussed in another section.

- The location of pes anserinus pain is more vague. It generally is located along the inner side of the back of the knee. This tendon runs along the inner knee below the joint line and can fan onto the upper leg bone just to the inside of the bony prominence at the top of the front of the leg bone, below the knee.

DESCRIPTION OF PAIN

- Popliteal pain is usually achy and felt deep in the area of the crease at the back of the knee. It often hurts after a workout, but may be present during it. There is often pain when the leg is extended and when pushing off. It may not hurt at rest.

- Medial hamstring tendinitis is noted by pain in the inside area of the back of the knee, along the tendon (can be felt when the knee is flexed). This pain can occur after a hard or fast workout or when walking fast on hilly terrain. It normally remains mild to moderate and hurts more when the leg is fully extended during gait. The tendon will often hurt when pressed.

- Pes anserinus pain is usually achy and noted on the inner side of the knee. It usually hurts at rest. After a few minutes of running/walking, the pain is often reduced. If the pain travels around to the front of the upper leg bone (tibia) it can be much more intense and cause limping in advanced cases, which can result in a compensation injury.

BASIC ANATOMY

- The pocket in the back of the knee is the popliteal fossa. Nerves, vessels, ligaments, and muscles cross through this area. First-time pain during or after a run/walk is almost always caused by the largest muscle in the pocket, the upper gastrocnemius (the upper calf muscle). Injury to this muscle is discussed in the calf pain section. Sometimes there is confusion as to the site of the injury because it may seem to come from lower thigh muscles.

- A Baker's cyst is a fluid-filled mass or lump that can appear in this pocket. This expansion from the knee joint sometimes protrudes into the upper gastrocnemius muscle. Internal knee irritation stimulates increased fluid inside the knee which is squeezed until it bulges backward into the fossa. The cyst can change in size from day to day.

- The inner margin of the popliteal fossa is formed by the medial (inner) hamstring tendon. Its job is to pull the lower leg back, or slow it down, as it straightens. It is heavily used during running and walking and is vulnerable to soreness with increases in speed or distance.

- Injury to the inner side of the knee and into the upper front of the leg bone is usually caused by the pes anserinus tendon and bursa. Pes anserinus means "goose's foot" in Greek—due to the shape of its three toes that are muscle tendons joining together. The larger single tendon formed by the junction wraps around the front of the leg bone and assists in bending and controlling the straightening of the leg. Its unique job is to rotate the leg bone. When the lower leg bone is rotating outward during the last few degrees of extension, this muscle pulls it back. It will also assist when the knee is rolling to the inside, as noticed in those with knock knees. A bursa is a fluid-filled sac of connective tissue that protects a tendon from rubbing excessively on a bone. If the pes anserinus experiences more rubbing that it can handle, it can damage the bursa that lies beneath it. This increases the fluid in the bursa, causing it to thicken, resulting in a painful condition called bursitis.

CAUSES

- The upper gastrocnemius muscle in the popliteal fossa is injured by excess stretching. Overzealous calf muscle stretching is the most common cause. Running on a surface that is too soft, or allowing the knee to straighten or become locked can aggravate it. Fast uphill walking, overstriding, and cycling can be causes.

- Baker's cysts within the fossa are caused by internal knee irritation. Sometimes this is due to irritation from a mileage or speed increase. Arthritis and meniscus tears can also be a cause.

- Medial hamstring tendon pain is caused by the same mechanisms as upper gastrocnemius pain, except calf stretching is not a cause.

- Pes anserinus pain is triggered by over extension of the leg, often due to overstriding and running faster. Excessive pronation and supination are strong contributors.

TREATMENT

- Icing is beneficial in treating all of these injuries.

- Slower, shorter workouts may allow for continued training; stay below the threshold of irritation.

- Upper gastrocnemius pain is reduced by adding heel lifts to shoes, cessation of stretching, taking strategic rest as needed, and avoiding hills. Physical therapy may be needed if the problem persists.

- Baker's cysts might indicate internal knee damage. A single episode of swelling in the popliteal fossa may mean that the knee became slightly aggravated during its adaptation. If the cyst persists or grows, see an orthopedist to ensure that this is not a more serious injury.

- Medial hamstring tendon pain will usually heal with decreased training, but if it persists, physical therapy can help. Overpronation or oversupination can also be a cause because the medial and lateral hamstrings may not be sharing the load evenly. Have your gait checked and get a shoe check from an experienced staff member at a technical running store.

- Pain along the inner knee at the joint line can be from pes anserinus tendinitis if there is diffuse soreness. Pain at the knee joint line that is more localized or is located slightly behind the knee can often turn out to be a meniscus tear inside the knee. If there is swelling with the pain, if it keeps recurring, or if it doesn't go away, have it evaluated by an orthopedist.

- The most common location for the pes anserinus injury is slightly below the knee joint line, with or without fanning onto the upper leg bone. Rest may be the only alternative if it becomes very sore. When there is bursitis, any activity will continue to aggravate the bursa. Shorten stride significantly, evaluate shoes and orthotics (looking at knee position more than foot position). If the knee is swinging toward the inside, a more stable shoe should be tried. With an outside swinging of the knee, a neutral or more cushioned shoe is possible. Don't massage because the bursa can be aggravated by aggressive rubbing. An elastic knee brace frequently helps. Physical therapy is often needed and a cortisone injection by an orthopedist should be considered. Bursitis is very responsive to injections. A single injection in this area is very conservative. An upper tibial stress fracture is a less common cause of pain in this area which can be determined by the orthopedist prior to the injection.

- Internal knee problems can be a cause if the knee feels irritated or is slow to heal. If you suspect this, see an orthopedist.

PEARLS

- Pes anserinus bursitis will stop an athlete from training immediately. Early treatment is important.

WHEN TO STOP TRAINING

- Most of these injuries are relatively mild and will permit training if diagnosed and treated early. One must stay below the threshold of irritation.

- Pes anserinus pain will continue to worsen if training continues once the pain reaches a stronger level.

CONSEQUENCES OF RUNNING OR WALKING THROUGH PAIN

- Generally, these injuries don't cause permanent damage. But other, more serious injuries could be present, which can compromise orthopedic health. Long-term training and racing with pain in this area is foolish. The pain could be due to a meniscus issue or stress fracture on the tibia inside the knee joint. But a single day of pushing through the pain is very unlikely to have permanent consequences.

ON THE OUTSIDE OF THE KNEE

ILIOTIBIAL BAND AND BICEPS FEMORIS INSERTION

LOCATION OF PAIN

- The pain is located on the outer knee. Pain in the outer thigh or hip is not included here.

- Iliotibial band (IT band) pain at the knee is sometimes hard to localize, but it is on the outer side of the knee. Sometimes it feels like pain is running down onto the outside and toward the front of the lower leg.

- Although the IT band is on the surface, sometimes IT band pain will feel internal. This is normal when it first occurs, but a doctor should be seen if it persists.

- Biceps femoris pain is felt toward the back of the knee. This is the tendon that comes out of the outside of the back of the thigh muscles (hamstrings). It can hurt in that area, and down to its insertion below the knee. The pain never moves towards the outside of the knee—only in back. Although biceps femoris and IT band pains feel similar, they require slightly different treatments. Strong IT band injury may include the biceps region, but the reverse is rarely true.

Iliotibial Band Syndrome

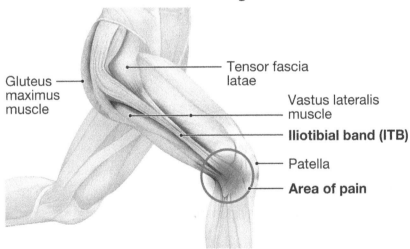

Gluteus maximus muscle

Tensor fascia latae

Vastus lateralis muscle

Iliotibial band (ITB)

Patella

Area of pain

DESCRIPTION OF PAIN

- IT band injury most commonly begins as an ache on the outside of the knee during a workout or race.

- If the pain continues to grow, it can become quite painful, making it difficult to flex the knee.

- Sometimes the first sensation occurs at the beginning of a short run after a longer or harder workout. This is because the damage can occur without pain, but is felt when the area is used again.

- Mild pain cannot be reproduced by pressing on the area. A more severe injury is indicated when you feel pain by pressing on it.

- The knee may not hurt with daily activity, although it may hurt for a day or two after a strong episode.

- Once injured, the IT band often begins hurting gradually during workouts. Only more advanced cases hurt from the start.

- Biceps femoris pain is similar, but less likely to become strong and more likely to grow gradually. BF pain is more likely with everyday activity, is present at the start of workouts, and decreases during shorter workouts.

BASIC ANATOMY

- The iliotibial band is a thick strand of connective tissue that begins as a muscle at the outer hip and continues as a strap of connective tissue that runs down the outer thigh and connects to the outside of the knee. The pain on the outer knee is discussed here.

- The IT band is tough connective tissue. Its job is to stabilize the knee when the foot is on the ground. If the knee moves in or out, it is stressed.

- The biceps femoris tendon attaches to the top of the outer lower leg bone (fibula). It travels behind the knee on the outside. It can easily be felt when the knee is flexed. Its job is to help flex the knee and slow it down when it is straightening. It is the connection point between the lower leg and the lateral hamstring muscles, the powerhouse of the hamstring group. When the knee is overextended, or pulls too hard against resistance, it becomes aggravated.

- Massaging the IT band above the knee is effective. Using a foam roller is an efficient way to achieve this. Jeff suggests rolling for 5 minutes before a run/walk, 5 minutes after a run/walk and 5 minutes before going to bed. There is less benefit from massage with a biceps femoris injury, but an experienced therapist can use special techniques that may speed up the healing process.

- IT band stretches can help recovery, but are valuable to prevent recurrences after the injury.

- Supination should be eliminated, and in fact temporary overpronation may be needed. Choose a shoe with more lateral motion control. If neutral cushioned shoes are already being used, consider a shoe in the lateral stability category or a trail shoe for roads since they usually have firmer outer edges to prevent ankle sprains, and the structure reduces stress on the lateral knee as the foot rolls forward. If it is obvious that overpronation is already present, or if you are experiencing other injuries such as medial shin pain, do not do this. Shoe experts in a technical running store can help you in choosing the right model.

- Avoid hills and faster running. Try to get a stride evaluation to identify causes such as overstriding. (Jeff conducts running form evaluations at his retreats and running schools).

- Elastic knee sleeves will sometimes help, and there are straps designed for IT band injuries that help mild injuries.

- When IT band injury is no longer present with daily activity after a rest period of two to three days, try a test run/walk. If there is immediate pain, stop. If it is comfortable, continue for 15 to 20 minutes only. If it begins to hurt before 20 minutes, stop. If 20 minutes is fine, wait a day to see if the pain increases afterward. If so, take another one to two days of rest/treatment and take a more liberal ratio of walking to running for 10 minutes. If the trial workout is successful, add a few minutes to the workout and try it again. Continue this progression, but if the injury returns, repeat the process. See a doctor if you have tried all of the treatments, and pain returns. It is best to run every other day and avoid any activity that could aggravate the injury.

NOTE: Jeff has had great success in returning clients to running by using liberal walk breaks from the beginning. He recommends starting back on the first run with a ratio of 10 to 15 seconds of running followed by 45 to 50 seconds of walking. With shorter running segments, the body can often continue to run, while the injury heals. See the section in this book on using the Run Walk Run method.

- A doctor will determine whether there is a more serious internal knee injury. A referral to a physical therapist can be very helpful. Sometimes an injection at the knee is performed. This is generally safe, but a high percentage of those injured are not helped by this. Due to the numbing from cortisone, one can aggravate the injury further without feeling the damage. An injection is best used when there is a lot of inflammation and it cannot be reduced through more conservative means. Through the years, IT band surgery has lost its popularity. It often was unsuccessful, and conservative therapy is effective but is slow.

- Orthotics designed by experienced doctors are helpful for difficult or repetitive injuries, but temporary versions add to the shoe changes for a single episode. Experienced staff members of running stores can help with the fitting issues because many orthotics make the injury worse. Incorporating a heel lift for a shorter leg should be included.

- Rest is always helpful, but with serious injuries it may take a long time to heal. Goals are often lost because of this injury, so early treatment is important. Jeff has found that when the run-walk-run ratio is conservative enough, most IT bands can heal while distance running is continued.

- Biceps femoris pain responds to these same treatments, but elevating both heels and immediately switching to trail shoes is advised.

PEARLS

- Many runners experience a strong pain during a workout, but it goes away quickly. However, many experience mild pain, and continue to train at the same level for weeks. The milder pain is easy to ignore and train, but running too hard with this condition can produce a long term injury. Short workouts and the right shoe can reduce this risk.

- The correct shoe can make a huge difference. It is common to feel fine in a shoe that causes the injury yet feel strange in the shoe that cures it.

- Many people need to overpronate a little permanently to prevent recurrent IT band irritation. Remember that changing the foot movement for even "normal feet" can be a cure for abnormal knees.

- Serious cases may require months to heal. Patience is required.

- Recurrent episodes can be eliminated, but many people require careful attention to all of the details to achieve results—especially more frequent walk breaks.

- Adaptation is necessary when a layoff of more than two months has occurred.

- Biceps femoris pain is often a singular problem and does not require adaptation.

- It is safe to carefully train with biceps femoris pain, but it may take a long time to go away. There are cases that require rest, but that is usually due to continuing to train at normal levels.

WHEN TO STOP TRAINING

- If possible, stop the workout as soon as IT band pain appears. Do not push through pain. A mild awareness is okay, but if it progresses, damage is progressing.

CONSEQUENCES OF RUNNING OR WALKING THROUGH PAIN

- IT band injury does not cause permanent damage, but it can take as long as a year to heal. If it occurs during an important race it may be worth the risk to finish. It often becomes impossible to maintain a normal stride, so important time goals are often not possible.

- Continuing to train with IT band pain is foolish. A very high percentage become so injured that extended rest is the only remedy.

UPPER LEG AND BUTT

ON THE INSIDE OF THE UPPER LEG—FROM THE GROIN OR LOWER BUTT MUSCLE IN THE DIRECTION OF THE KNEE

MEDIAL THIGH PAIN

LOCATION OF PAIN

- This pain can originate as high as the upper groin area and sometimes on the hard bone that is felt when sitting on a hard surface near the inner side of each gluteal area. It travels downward along the inner side of the thigh, but usually there is no pain near the knee.

DESCRIPTION OF PAIN

- Running and walking produce a different kind of injury than that caused by lateral-movement sports unless the injury arises from sprinting, weightlifting, or stretching. Runners and walkers usually experience a slow increase in pain, on the inner side of the thigh, during a workout or over several workouts.

- If the pain begins suddenly without a noticeable cause, such as tripping or jumping over an object, it would be wise to see a doctor. Particularly seek treatment if the pain is high up in the groin or toward the hip. (This can be a stress fracture, hernia, or a nerve injury, among other injuries.)

- If the pain begins suddenly, even when caused by a known reason, and persists with rest, it is also wise to see a doctor.

- The more common type of running/walking medial thigh injury is a low grade ache that often warms up and goes away within the first few minutes of a workout. It may return toward the end if the workout is long. It is easily aggravated by faster running, downhill running, and some feel that cold weather aggravates the symptoms.

BASIC ANATOMY

- The medial thigh has a group of muscles called the adductors that sometimes are called groin muscles. These muscles pull the legs toward each other, especially when the knees are not bent. They are stretched when the legs are spread.

- The adductors are also stretched when the stride is longer than the length that is natural for the individual.

- They originate from several places on the pelvis. These are very weak attachments. The bone connections are easily injured.

- These narrow, long muscles heal very slowly.

CAUSES

- These muscles gradually grow stronger as training progresses. Sometimes they are not able to handle the increase and become sore. Slight soreness is normal, especially when in both legs. Continuing to increase intensity or endurance is a mistake because the muscles are relatively fragile.

- Sudden extension of the stride or a rapid side step can injure them, but usually the injury occurs gradually.

- Weight-training on a machine that squeezes the knees together from a spread leg position can cause this injury.

- Overstretching is a cause, and stretching this area with a fresh injury is very likely to cause progression of the injury.

TREATMENT

- Stop stretching the area.

- Ice massage.

- Take a few days off from running (3-5 days).

- Make sure there is not too much supination or that the shoes are not too worn.

- If the pain persists, physical therapy can help.

- If the pain is high in the groin and into the pelvic area and does not improve with rest, see a doctor.

- Ask your doctor if prescription strength anti-inflammatory medication can help.

- There are several serious injuries in this area that should be ruled out or diagnosed.

PEARLS

- If the pain is lower, in the middle of the thigh, is mild, yet seems to be lasting for weeks, there may be no long-term harm to running/walking conservatively without increased mileage. These injuries often take several months to heal, regardless of treatment.

WHEN TO STOP TRAINING

- A few days off for healing in the early stages of an injury can reduce the time off from running dramatically.

CONSEQUENCES OF RUNNING OR WALKING THROUGH PAIN

- Finishing a race is okay unless the pain is very strong near the pelvis. We have seen a significant number of stress fractures at the femoral neck that require surgery if they progress. If runners insert recovery and rest early, only crutches are needed. This often happens in ONE event, with no previous pain.

- As mentioned, many people elect to train very conservatively with mild lower adductor injuries. But if they push too hard, the pain can move up to the origin and become a much more serious injury.

OUTSIDE OF THE THIGH GOING DOWN FROM THE BONY KNOB ON THE OUTSIDE OF THE HIP

LATERAL THIGH PAIN

LOCATION OF PAIN

- This includes pain in the thigh from the bony knob on the outside of the hip, about four or five inches below the waist, down to the tendon of the iliotibial band. It does not include pain behind or in front of the hip knob.

DESCRIPTION OF PAIN

- This pain is diffuse and achy except for that coming from the hip bone knob. That pain can be focused, deeply sore, and sometimes fairly sharp. Pain on the knob can also result in a clicking or popping sensation once it is inflamed.

BASIC ANATOMY

- The broad fleshy muscle on the outside of the hip has a thin tough layer of connective tissue that lies on the outside. Starting from the waist, this band narrows gradually and passes over the outer hip knob—a protruding bump from the hip bone (femur) called the greater trochanter. A bursa between the muscle and the greater trochanter is supposed to protect the muscle from irritation by the greater trochanter. The bursa is a fluid-filled connective tissue sack that sometimes becomes irritated, a condition called bursitis.

- As the fleshy muscle passes down below the greater trochanter, it blends with the iliotibial tract. This is a flat strap of connective tissue that continues down to the knee.

CAUSES

- Upper thigh pain is caused by extra tension on the fleshy muscle area against the greater trochanter. This is especially common when people sag into their hips and tilt when they absorb impact during gait. Wide hips, crossover gait, too much supination, training on a slanted surface, and having one leg longer than the other are causes. Less commonly, strong overpronation may produce irritation when the knees move together.

- Lateral thigh pain is almost always caused by too much supination. It is normal to get sore in this area when running downhill, increasing mileage, and when running fast workouts. If the pain is increasing or is very strong, seek treatment.

- In rare situations, nerve injury, such as from the lower back, can be a cause.

TREATMENT

- Ice, decreased mileage, and a permanent or a temporary quarter-inch heel lift on the opposite side are treatments. The lift becomes permanent if it is determined that your longer leg is on the sore side. If the pain lingers or the injury reoccurs, strengthening the gluteal muscles can help decrease the sinking or dropping of the hip during gait. Physical therapy is helpful, and a cortisone injection is rarely required. Sometimes running form improvement can stop the sinking of the hips. In many cases, the body adapts and the problem goes away.

- If the lateral thigh is more sore than would be expected from normal hard training, decreasing supination usually helps. Less stable shoes and custom medical orthotics can help. Orthotics should be crafted by a person experienced in sports injuries. Poorly made orthotics can make the situation worse. Massage to the lateral thigh or use of a foam roller is very helpful. Do not massage or roll the greater trochanter area as this can irritate the bursa.

PEARLS

- Often the pain is first noticed while sleeping on the sore side.

- Women develop hip pain more than men. Pregnancies can increase the symptoms, as can carrying a child on the same side—even when it is noticed during workouts.

- If the greater trochanteric bursitis pain is strong, it may take months to heal.

- Pain that includes the knob on the upper hip and deeper areas nearby can be early stage hip arthritis, especially if there is a decrease in the "hip in and out" rotation range or "reduced rotation" pain. The knob itself is not part of the hip joint. The actual joint begins deeper near the knob.

WHEN TO STOP TRAINING

- It is possible to train through mild versions of these injuries, but pain at the greater trochanter should be monitored.

- If greater trochanteric bursitis is serious, it is almost impossible for it to heal while continuing to work out.

CONSEQUENCES OF RUNNING ORWALKING THROUGH PAIN

- A single day of running/walking through the pan is unlikely to have long-term effect, but ignoring upper greater trochanteric hip pain could require months to heal.

FROM THE UPPER BUTT MUSCLE DOWN THE BACKSIDE OF THE UPPER LEG TO THE KNEE

HAMSTRING PAIN

LOCATION OF PAIN

- Pain often starts in lower pelvic bone called the ischial tuberosity. When the hip is flexed repeatedly, this area gets irritated and hurts. Nerves can also become irritated, sending pain down the hamstring muscle toward the knee. Many hamstring injuries hurt only on the ischial tuberosity.

- Most commonly when running/walking, the pain will be along the back of the thigh.

- Pain above the bony ischial tuberosity is not a hamstring injury.

- Pain that includes the hamstrings and the area above the ischial tuberosity should be treated as a hip/gluteal injury with the possibility of a back injury.

DESCRIPTION OF PAIN

- Runners/walkers often notice this first during a run, or shortly afterward, in the middle portion of the back of the thigh. This is usually a mildly achy deep soreness.

- The pain may feel like it has healed when walking around during daily activities, but reappear during a run. Fatigue, faster running, and hills will aggravate the hamstring.

- If the pain is on the ischial tuberosity, it can be mildly achy to quite sore. Severe cases may prevent sitting and cause discomfort while driving.

- Sudden onset of strong pain is less common during running/walking unless sprinting or taking a sudden extended movement of the leg. This type of injury can leave the area mildly sore for a few days, with some limping. Severe cases require the use of crutches, and produce noticeable bruising and swelling in the muscles—occasionally a rupture. In this case, see a doctor.

- Pain that includes the hip above the ischial tuberosity and the hamstrings is often related to nerve injury. The pain will be along a long portion of the

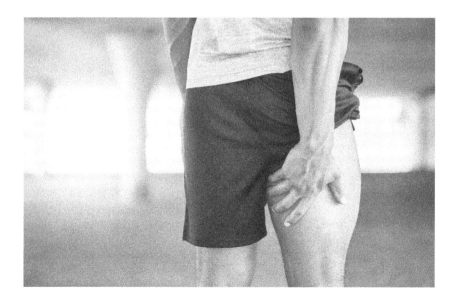

muscle and difficult to define. Sitting and particularly driving may irritate the injury. If the hamstring pain continues below the knee, it is almost certainly related to the nerve.

BASIC ANATOMY

- There are three long muscles that originate at the ischial tuberosity and travel down the back of the thigh attaching below the knee, on the back and inside portion of the upper leg bone. One of these muscles has a second muscle mass that originates from the back of the thigh bone itself. They join together and become one strand called the biceps femoris.

- These muscles extend across two joints—the hip and the knee—and have many possible areas of irritation. As the knee extends to its almost straight position, the muscle contracts to control and restrain the forward momentum. This type of contraction is stressful to muscles. At this moment, the position of the hip will influence the length of the muscle. The muscles in the front of the thigh (quadriceps) are pulling the knee into a straightened position with great force, while the hamstrings oppose this motion with less strength. The greater the range of motion, the greater the stress.

- Hamstring injuries most commonly occur at the ischial tuberosity or at various places in the muscle strands—usually in the middle. Sometimes the bone can be injured, which can take a long time to heal. Where the muscle connects to the ischial tuberosity there is also a bursa, which is a fluid filled sack of connective tissue protecting the hamstring. Bursitis at this spot is common.

CAUSES

- The most common cause is continuing to run and walk after the muscle has become extremely fatigued. Muscles will work until they are so weakened and irritated that they suffer tears in the areas that are overworked. Gradual and regular increases in workload, with rest in between, stimulates the tendons, muscles, and their origins to grow stronger, adapting to more stress.

- Overstretching is a common cause—especially when the hamstring is fatigued or has become irritated. During one stretching session the pain can move from a milder middle muscle soreness to a serious ischial tuberosity injury.

- Overstriding, especially with the pelvis rotated forward, is a very common cause. Strong stomach muscles keep the pelvis straightened and the ischial tuberosity slightly closer to the knee. There is less stress on the hamstrings in this position.

- Weak hamstrings relative to the quadriceps (front thigh muscles) can put more demand on the hamstrings.

- If the hamstrings are very tight, there can be more stress. This is not usually a problem for recreational runners who don't do speedwork or lateral motion sports, and keep the stride short.

- Chronic hamstring injuries are caused by all of the above, but scars from past injuries can develop, preventing normal function of the muscle.

TREATMENT

- Mild pain may be healed during a couple of rest days. Icing is useful. Do not stretch. Massage can be very helpful, especially if the pain lasts more than a couple of days. The foam roller and "the stick" are good modes of treatment.

- Start all runs with a 3- to 5-minute gentle walk. Avoid hills. Gradually introduce the body to running with 10 to 60 seconds of running, alternating with 60 seconds of walking.

- If the injury persists and the problem is still in the middle of the muscle, or if the pain is fairly strong, see a doctor. Physical therapy modalities can help, especially a focused manual therapy technique (various types should be used).

- If the pain is at the ischial tuberosity, icing is more difficult but still helps. Massage can be beneficial if you don't have a bursitis (massage may make it worse). Massage is actually a good diagnosis technique to determine if you have a bursitis or not. A steroid injection may help a bursitis. Injecting other hamstring conditions is not recommended. There are special cushions available that make sitting less irritating.

- In serious cases, extended time off from running may be required. During this time, water running can maintain a great deal of the running adaptations, and careful strengthening of the hamstring should help. If a given form of exercise produces more soreness, try other exercises. Cycling can be beneficial: The front thigh muscles are used a great deal in cycling, but the hamstrings get some gentle exercise. Make sure the seat is high enough to engage the hamstrings. Ride in an easy gear until the pain has improved. For long-term benefit the effort level needs to be significant and not just pedaling easily. Spinning classes on a stationary bike can be helpful, also climbing hills while cycling. Cycling can be continued for as long as the pain continues and longer for prevention of future problems.

- Chronic hamstring injuries don't tend to heal with normal amounts of rest; the pain may go away for a while and then keep coming back. This indicates that the hamstrings did not have enough time to heal or there were excessive demands on them, too soon, during the return to running. To heal the hamstrings properly, it may be necessary to use several approaches at one time: 1) Strengthening of the gluteal muscles and the abdominal muscles. 2) Massage by a practitioner who has had plenty of experience treating athletes. 3) Completely evaluating the structure of the feet, legs, and hips for symmetry and motion. 4) Evaluate the stride for proper body position. There are many sources of advice on proper stride, but pelvic position should be checked. When standing against a wall, the lower back, just above the waist, should be flattened against the wall without leaning away from the wall. If this is not happening, tighten abdominal muscles. Trying to maintain this pelvic position while running/walking decreases the stretch on the hamstrings, and provides other valuable benefits. Modalities using electrical current and other devices have been helpful to heal resistant cases. Stretching prescribed by a trained medical practitioner can be useful—but be careful.

- Very resistant cases can take months to a year to heal.

PEARLS

- There are encouraging reports of other potential treatments: high-intensity shock treatment to the ischial tuberosity, acupuncture, laser, topical creams such as Arnica and Voltaren, unique exercises like running backward to retrain the muscles, and various taping methods.

- Elastic thigh sleeves help some athletes.

- Automobiles with low seats can aggravate an injury.

- Subtle imbalances in the gluteal muscles and back muscles can lead to nerve irritation that predisposes the hamstrings to injury.

WHEN TO STOP TRAINING

- Commonsense test workouts after a short period of rest can give a reality check. Many athletes try to continue to train, ignoring the pain. In the early stages, many hamstring injuries remain only moderately painful and allow for continued training. But continued running can aggravate the injury significantly, requiring months to heal (as opposed to days or weeks when healed early). It is best to err on the side of rest when the injury first occurs.

CONSEQUENCES OF RUNNING OR WALKING THROUGH PAIN

- Hamstring cramping can occur in long events and feel like an injury. Achy muscular soreness can occur in hard events or fast workouts. It is generally safe to continue if almost normal gait is possible. Heavy limping and stronger pain may represent a more serious injury and further damage can result. Stop running and walk if the injury occurred during a workout.

FRONT OF THE HIP, JUST ABOVE OR JUST BELOW WHERE THE LEG ATTACHES JUST ABOVE OR JUST BELOW

HIP FLEXOR INJURY

LOCATION OF PAIN

- The pain is located in the soft tissue at the front of the hip on or just below the bony knob in the front of the hip bone. This is just below the belt line in front. It may spread down onto the uppermost part of the thigh as well.

- When the hip is flexed, as when sitting, and the leg is lifted, the pain should be in the fleshy tendon and muscle mass that tightens just below the bony bump on the hip in front. It may hurt on the bump itself.

DESCRIPTION OF PAIN

- During a run/walk the pain usually comes on gradually. First symptoms are usually an achy feeling as the leg is extended behind and as it comes forward. This is followed by stiffness and soreness after the workout, after sitting, and in the morning after waking. Many experience pain when getting in or out of a car.

- The pain starts out dull, but may become sharp as damage increases.

- In the beginning stages, most runners experience minimal pain. If ignored, the injury can progress and force one to limp.

- If there is pain is on the knob of bone at the hip, it may be sharply painful from the beginning. This can become a long-term injury and should be treated immediately.

- It will often hurt after sitting when the leg is raised and the hip is flexed.

- Sometimes the pain occurs suddenly due to an unexpected motion like tripping. It is common in other sports with fast lateral movements. It can easily be injured in stretching or other exercises including weight lifting (often due initially to over stretching the hip). These rapid onset injuries may be quite painful. If experiencing serious pain, see a doctor.

BASIC ANATOMY

- Three hip flexor muscles are primarily responsible for moving the thigh upward and help initiate the pull of the leg forward when it is fully extended to the rear.

- The rectus femoris is a quadriceps muscle from the front of the thigh that attaches to the bone at the hip in front. Injury to this muscle causes pain at the upper portion of the thigh and is one of two primary muscles causing pain near the bone on the front of the hip. The sartorius is connected to the bump itself and wraps to the inside of the thigh. Sartorius is not one of the primary hip flexors but is affected by the way the hip extends and flexes.

- There are two muscles that originate at the front of the lower back and deep in the pelvis. These are the iliacus and psoas major. They are sometimes called the iliopsoas. They travel down and forward to attach to the hipbone on the inner and back just below the hip joint. Because they wrap around the bone, they also rotate the thigh outward as they lift it upward.

- If the pain is on the inner portion of the muscle and tendon mass, and hurts when raising the leg while sitting (with the knee straightened), the primary muscle suspect is the iliopsoas.

- There is a fluid filled bursa that will sometimes become sore and inflamed in this area.

- Some people notice a snapping of the tendon when the hip is twisted and moved forward and backward in the front of the hip. This usually does not cause pain.

- There are a number of other reasons for deeper pain in this area including hernias, stress fractures, and damage to the joint. If the problem does not follow the typical pattern mentioned here, it is wise to see a doctor.

CAUSES

- Sitting for long hours during the workday reduces flexibility in the hip flexor region. Many runners have weak abdominal muscles which puts extra stress on this area. The hip flexors can be easily overwhelmed and injured during longer runs or walks due to the extension of the hip joint as the legs move forward and backward repeatedly.

- Running or walking faster (than in the recent past) forces the leg to extend farther to the rear. This is normal but until the body properly adapts, it can irritate this area.

- Lifting the leg farther than normal, repeatedly, is also a cause. This occurs when running uphill, during speedwork, and when racing.

- This injury is more likely when the pelvis is tilted forward. Since two of the primary muscles originate within the pelvis, it's important that it be aligned properly.

- Excessive pronation, and less commonly supination, can force the leg to move forward and backward with more of a circular motion. This twists the hip slightly and can aggravate and pull the muscles and tendons diagonally. This is also a common cause of pain on the bone bump at the front of the hip.

- Stretching is a common cause of hip flexor injury. Too much work in hip strength exercises can also be a cause.

TREATMENT

- Icing, massage, and initial rest.

- Massage is often painful when done correctly by an experienced therapist, but it can speed the healing. The pain usually goes away after the treatment.

- Stretching should be avoided until after the injury has been in a healing mode. It is best used, carefully, to prevent recurrence.

- Evaluate the gait for overpronation and supination as well as inefficient running form.

- If the problem persists or is very painful, see a doctor. The more serious pain can indicate a joint problem or a bone injury among other issues.

- Physical therapy may be needed if pain persists. Electrical modalities, manual therapy, and peripheral muscle strengthening is helpful.

- This injury can last for many months, especially if it is ignored, and training is continued with pain.

- An MRI can define which tissue is injured and sometimes locate scarring on the tendon. Diagnostic injection can sometimes be productive when performed by a skilled sports orthopedist. Ask the doctor why extended rest is needed, if this is prescribed.

PEARLS

- With mild cases, a couple of days of rest and icing can usually get the healing started. Training is usually possible afterward if one stays below the threshold of further irritation.

- When there is a recurrent or difficult problem, a good physical therapy package should involve extensive evaluation of the hip to investigate why there is extra stress on the hip flexors.

- Continuous pain that does not seem to heal after extensive conservative care often turns out to be arthritis. Decreased ability to turn the hip in or out is a clue.

WHEN TO STOP TRAINING

- Early rest is recommended, but if the problem persists or mistakes were made in the early stages, extended rest may be the only way to avoid pain.

- Many runners have trained through months of pain in this area. This often increases the time needed for healing. Even if there is no increase in pain or injury, it is wise to get a good diagnosis. Cease training if there is significant pain or the pain increases. Continuous irritation of a tendon can cause it to develop a form of scarring called tendinosis that is very difficult to heal. Other therapies can be performed during this time to improve the healing process. Some of these are risky and should be considered carefully.

CONSEQUENCES OF RUNNING OR WALKING THROUGH PAIN

- Ignoring the pain and avoiding treatment can increase the damage and create a resistant long-term problem. Competitive athletes may need at least a year, in many cases, to get back to previous conditioning.

BUTT MUSCLE PAIN FROM THE WAIST TO THE LOWER FOLD IN THE BUTT

GLUTEAL PAIN AND PIRIFORMIS SYNDROME

LOCATION OF PAIN

- This "pain in the butt" can be located below the waist down to the fold where the gluteus muscles meet the back of the thigh. Laterally, it can hurt anywhere from the outer hip bone (greater trochanter) to the tail bone.

DESCRIPTION OF PAIN

- Commonly there is a deep, achy pain that sometimes spreads downward into the back of the thigh. It can originate from the area behind the outer hip bone (greater trochanter) toward the middle of the gluteal area. It rarely becomes a sharper pain.

- It will hurt during training and afterward. Sitting can aggravate it.

- It usually begins gradually and is mild enough to ignore at first. If not treated it can progress and hurt in every workout, but is worse during hill runs and long runs/walks.

- The pain is sometimes hard to pinpoint and may move a little each day.

- It hurts more when pressing firmly with the fingers deeply into the gluteal area. Rubbing or massaging the area may provide relief.

- Stretching the hip by turning the leg outward or inward may either provide relief or stimulate the pain.

- Another variation is pain felt near the waist or streaks of pain going into the thigh and sometimes the lower leg. See a doctor in these cases to investigate nerve symptoms from the back or other areas. The pain may come from the spine even when not felt in the back.

BASIC ANATOMY

- Most commonly, the pain comes from one or more of the gluteal muscle groups.

- There are also six smaller muscles in the area, and it is often difficult to pinpoint the source—which is not needed for prescribing treatment. Conservative treatment and the treatment listed below works for all muscle groups.

- The sciatic nerve passes through this area and can be irritated by the muscles when they tighten.

- Piriformis syndrome is the common name for pain deep in the gluteal area. Although it is suspected that the piriformis muscle is the most common source of this pain, it is hard to prove. A deep nerve pain which may radiate often indicates piriformis involvement. The piriformis muscle sits against the sciatic nerve in a variety of ways that make it susceptible to aggravation. Muscle action (rubbing and tightening) can irritate the sciatic nerve producing nerve pain.

- If the pain is higher in the gluteal area, but below the waist by a couple of inches, especially toward the outer half, it is probably a gluteal injury and not the classic piriformis syndrome.

- If the pain is on the prominent bone that is felt when sitting on a hard surface (ischial tuberosity), the origin of the pain is often from the thigh muscles (hamstrings or adductors) and not related to this injury.

- It is wise to seek medical help if the pain seems unusual, strong, or occurs without a logical reason; there could be more serious conditions that should be investigated.

CAUSES

- A repetitive outward turning motion of the hip is the most common cause. When the thigh bone turns out, forcing the knee to point out, these muscles are stressed. This occurs more on uphills, when running faster, and when extending stride length when either running or walking. The motion may be very subtle and one is often unaware it is happening. When the foot is planted, the outward twist or torque force is absorbed by the pelvis because the leg and the foot are locked as a unit to the ground. As the heel leaves the ground, the extra thrust that pushes the other hip forward comes from a team effort of the calf muscles and the rotation muscles at the hip, including the piriformis. Any of these can become sore and injured. As noted, hill running, longer strides, and faster propulsion will increase the need for an extra thrust and result in more aggravation.

- Sitting for long periods can irritate these muscles.

- The sensitive deeper muscles work harder when the bigger gluteal muscles are weak.

- Inefficient running form or alignment can increase the irritation. The forwardly rotated pelvis can be a source of this, as mentioned in the hamstring injury section.

- Excessive pronation causes the foot to roll too far inward, rotating the leg and hip inward. This forces the hip muscles to pull harder to resupinate the foot at push-off. If the excess pronation forces the knee to rotate inward, the gluteal muscles can be irritated due to overstretching.

- If the piriformis muscle is inflamed, overdeveloped and enlarged from repetitive use, or stretched excessively against the sciatic nerve, there can be nerve irritation (sciatica). This can produce a variety of symptoms that may or may not radiate down the leg.

- Lateral pain that is higher in the gluteal area can have the same cause, but it is most commonly due to stepping up or sinking into the hip (noted by the other hip dropping below the level of the standing one). The stepping up occurs when climbing, and the sinking will occur while compensating for unequal leg lengths, weak gluteal muscles, and striking the ground with higher impact. Increased impact can come from overstriding, particularly when running downhill, meaning that the leg is landing with the knee locked straight. In this case, the hip absorbs the impact usually accepted by the thigh muscles (when the knee is slightly flexed).

- Lack of flexibility in the hip muscles may be a cause, but less often. Some studies show that women are five times more likely than men to suffer this injury, which may indicate that lack of strength may be part of the problem. Extreme tightness can be a cause, but it is unlikely that moderate tightness is as much of a problem as muscle weakness.

- Many people experience a torque or a turning of the pelvis. This can be from previous injury, compensation for a leg length difference, asymmetric strength, and sometimes genetic issues. In each case, extra stress is absorbed by the gluteal and deeper muscles.

TREATMENT

- Most athletes will experience short periods of soreness in this area which is of little concern. A couple of days of rest from the offending motion will allow for healing. If not responsive, or if it keeps reoccurring, additional treatment should be used. This is a deep injury, so a longer recovery time is advised. If there is surface inflammation, use ice. If the muscle swells, it may irritate the nerve. Massage is almost always helpful.

- Get a shoe check to ensure that you are receiving the needed stability to control or eliminate overpronation. Consider a gait analysis to note running form irregularities. Gentle stretching of the hip may help, but be careful. This means both inwardly and outwardly rotating the thigh bone in the hip joint. When doing this, get instruction from a professional. Do not stretch or rotate into pain of any type.

- If the pain persists, an evaluation of the hip should be considered, especially if there is any radiation of the pain downward or upward toward the lower back or tailbone. This can be done by a doctor so that other medical reasons can be eliminated or diagnosed. An X-ray is helpful to rule out hip, joint, and back problems. If nerve pain is the primary symptom, an MRI is a good idea. These are not very effective for diagnosing muscular pain, however.

- Physical therapy is the most effective treatment for this problem. An evaluation of the back, hip position, muscular strength and flexibility, unequal leg length, and related weakness such as abdominal strength, might be necessary to construct a rehabilitation program. More difficult cases require addressing each of these. Manual therapy is very useful, and can help to straighten a rotated pelvis. A comprehensive PT program can also apply specific massage techniques to improve muscle function and healing. This often involves strengthening the uninjured hip muscles.

- Extreme cases may require injections by an orthopedist, with mixed results. Recent evidence indicates that in certain cases Botox injections can atrophy the muscle and relieve pressure on the nerve to reduce the random and excessive firing, but long-term effects are not known.

PEARLS

- This injury can be persistent.

- It may occur in beginners, but a high percentage of victims are experienced athletes who are increasing volume or changing terrain.

- Some women experience this pain during pregnancy, and it goes away after the child is born.

- The pain is often experienced in glute on the shorter leg side, but some of the shortening may be due to the injury itself (from hip rotation). A manual therapy practitioner can often determine if this is the cause, and a heel lift can be a form of treatment.

- If sitting irritates the area, a special cushion can be purchased. To test the need, try sitting on a small soft pillow under one hip at a time. Sometimes it feels best under the sore hip and other times under the painless side.

WHEN TO STOP TRAINING

- Because the symptoms are mild at first, it is easy to ignore a gluteus injury until it has progressed. Even if it is mild enough to tolerate and rest helped a little, do not ignore it. Use the treatments mentioned until symptoms disappear. If the pain increases or does not seem to be improving steadily stop training for a few days.

- If it persists and becomes very painful, rest will be needed along with rehabilitation treatment.

CONSEQUENCES OF RUNNING OR WALKING THROUGH PAIN

- A single event or workout may be the cause. Even when there is strong pain, you may recover in a couple of days. In other cases with the same symptoms, more rest is needed. Use common sense but it is usually safe to finish an easy run. Limping or sharp piercing pain is a signal to stop.

- Continuing to train is risky. If the diagnosis has been confirmed and other reasons for the pain are eliminated as causes, runners will sometimes recover while significantly reducing the weekly mileage and intensity. Significant injury can result if the sciatic nerve symptoms are ignored and the potential for a long healing process is likely. The muscles can develop scarring and fibrosis as well, and compensating for the injury can result in an injury that is much worse.

THE BACK

VARIOUS PROBLEMS IN THE LOWER BACK

LOWER BACK PAIN

LOCATION OF PAIN

- Various pains that originate above the waist (or anywhere along the midline of the back) down to the tailbone below the waist. Pain may also extend away from this area.

- Sometimes it is only on the outer side of the lower back above the waist.

DESCRIPTION OF PAIN

- The pain on the outer sides of the lower back may feel achy and inside the muscles. It may occur after a hard or longer run, after running hills. It may be on one or both sides.

- Sometimes the back will feel stiff. Other times it will feel achy. Pain may become sharp or feel like a muscle spasm. A deep burning has been described as well.

- Sometimes the pain only occurs after working out. Other times it hurts with daily activity. If it hurts during workouts, it is usually progressing and getting a bit worse.

- The first symptoms occur the morning after a hard workout, making it difficult to get out of bed.

BASIC ANATOMY

- The back is complex and difficult to diagnose when injured.

- It is difficult to determine whether it is nerve irritation or simple muscle pain.

- Pain toward the outer back is more likely to be muscular.

CAUSES

- Mild back soreness related to a hard workout or change in terrain is common.

- Posture and running form is a very common cause. Pelvic rotation as mentioned in the hamstring section is a trigger for either mild nerve pain or muscular pain.

- Unequal leg length and a torqued or turned pelvis is a cause.

- A significant number of people develop changes in the bones of the spine that increase the pain. This can be arthritis.

- Weak muscles, particularly in the abdominal region, can be a strong contributor.

TREATMENT

- Mild muscle pain will get better with rest. Ice and massage help.

- If the pain is stronger or persists, see a doctor.

- X-rays can tell if the nerves are affected or if the shape of the spine is normal. They are not always conclusive, but they can usually highlight serious problems. If the X- rays are fairly normal, conservative treatment usually works.

- As long as it does not irritate the problem area, begin abdominal strengthening.

- Evaluate shoes for stability and gait for correct form.

- Seek help from a doctor sooner rather than later for back problems. Getting an early and accurate diagnosis can prevent needless aggravation and wasted time. The back is injured often and there are a lot of treatments available.

- Physical therapy with an emphasis on manual techniques is nearly always beneficial.

- Specific strengthening exercises may help, and perhaps stretching (often you will not stretch the back itself). Get guidance from a specialist before stretching.

- Surgery should be avoided unless years of conservative treatment has failed. Other treatments such as injections are much safer. It is best to know why surgery is the best and only option.

PEARLS

- For mild arthritic changes, mild disc problems, and recurrent muscular injury, core muscle strengthening, proper form, and correct shoes can help.

- Many runners with more severe arthritis and damage in the back are able to continue pain free by incorporating run-walk-run ratios.

- For persistent problems that are not caused by significant changes in the back bones, yoga over a long period of time has proven useful. This must be done carefully and with the advice of the person supervising the physical therapy portion of the treatment.

- Many people have had to stop running because of back problems, but some have stopped too soon when a thorough rehabilitation program could have eliminated their pain.

WHEN TO STOP TRAINING

- Back pain is often a deteriorating condition. If the pain is slight, and lasts a few days, a careful decrease in mileage and a few days of rest will eliminate the symptoms. Continue training if the injury only appears intermittently and shows mild symptoms. Be sure to start strengthening the abdominal muscles, get a shoe check at a technical running store, and improve form. As long as the episodes become further apart and eventually go away, it is fine to continue training.

- If the pain spreads or worsens, stop training and get help.

CONSEQUENCES OR RUNNING OR WALKING THROUGH PAIN

- Mild to moderate back pain during a workout or race is common. It is usually safe to finish.

- Any back pain that makes it hard to run or especially walk without limping is a reason to stop training.

- Even if you have been able to continue running with pain, the limping motion will eventually cause something else to become injured.

OVER-THE-COUNTER DRUG ISSUES

NON-STEROIDAL ANTI-INFLAMMATORY MEDICATION (NSAID)

USE IN SPORTS INJURIES

NSAIDS are a class of medications we know as over-the-counter pain pills. Although there are prescription versions which are not over-the-counter, they are similar. These can be ibuprofen, naproxen, aspirin, ketoprofen, celecoxib, piroxicam, salsalate, and diclofenac as well as many others. These names are the generic names and not the brand names, so there are many versions with different brand names (such as Advil, Nuprin, and Naprosyn) for each of these as well.

Acetaminophen—also known as Tylenol, has different characteristics, treats pain, but does not prevent inflammation—is not included in this classification, and there are natural pain relievers that are also not in this class such as Arnica.

They have been recommended for years to treat injuries. The theory was that the beginning of an injury is accompanied by inflammation. This is a process by the body to handle the trauma of tissue damage. It involves releasing chemicals that cause swelling, pain, production of cells that absorb damaged tissue, and increasing the blood flow. It was assumed that this process, although normal, needs to be finished before the true repair process could begin. It was often assumed that the body tends to exceed what is necessary to begin the healing process and it would be a benefit to shorten the duration of inflammation and minimize the amount of inflammation so overall healing is faster.

The NSAIDS block the inflammation process. Each has a slightly different mechanism and strength, but their primary job is to interfere with the process of allowing the inflammation to continue. Intuitively, since pain is decreased as inflammation is decreased, we tend to think the result is a benefit. It is a benefit if the goal is only to reduce pain. The problem is that good research has caused us to question our conclusions. Studies have shown delayed healing of bone injuries, surgical wounds, tendon connection to bone, tendons, and muscles when NSAIDS are used. These studies have also shown decreased response to training in muscles so that the process of growing stronger through exercise is slowed.

NSAIDS also have been associated with other side effects: gastric ulcers, increased blood pressure, gastric bleeding, and kidney problems, and has been connected with serious sodium problems especially when athletes are dehydrated as in a long race. These side effects occur even with fairly small doses and without long-term use.

There have been several cases of hyponatremia in marathons that were directly linked to the ingestion of NSAIDS before or during a marathon. We advise not taking these medications during or before any event lasting more than three hours.

So, the benefits of using NSAIDS are possibly decreased pain, less muscle soreness during a hard event (although the actual muscle damage is not reduced), and less soreness after a hard event (but studies show no faster recovery and some suggest it delays recovery); theoretically if you are going to work out on an injured body part, even though you know it is damaged, it may do less harm if the tissue is not inflamed during the work out.

Many people have taken these medications by doctor's suggestion when they are injured and the injury has healed. Good studies have shown that for the types of injuries most runners and walkers develop, the injury heals whether the medication is taken or not and it did not affect the healing. It just healed while the NSAID was being taken. This was shown using placebos.

At the present time it is advisable to avoid NSAIDS for treating these common injuries because although the risks are small on a statistical basis, the actual benefits do not outweigh the risks. There are other ways to decrease the mild to moderate pain usually caused by these injuries. Think of this tolerable pain as a good thing because the body's healing process is in action. For stronger pain and especially if prescribed by a doctor (there are other reasons NSAIDS are prescribed), the balance tips in favor of the benefits of taking them.

As in other medical issues, our best advice is that you get the best advice you can from a doctor who knows your medical history and wants you to have a long running life.

PHYSICAL THERAPY

In the treatment sections, the term *physical therapy* is used. This is a description of treatment that is provided by several medical specialties. It can be manual therapy with special massage and range of motion techniques including manipulation. Other modalities include ultrasound, muscle stimulation, laser, acupuncture with and without stimulation, and other forms of electric and magnetic applications. PT treatments also include stretching, strengthening, balance exercises, and the formulation of home exercise plans.

Physical therapy can be performed by practitioners called physical therapists, but it can also be performed by others. Examples are chiropractors, athletic trainers, podiatrists, nurses, and medical doctors (orthopedists and physiatrists, most commonly). These practitioners have a license that is required for most of the modalities. Acupuncture is performed by practitioners called acupuncturists, but some of these other professions become trained and include it in their practices. Some specialists use all of these treatments and some may feature only a few.

It is important to know that the name of the profession is not as important as the skill and experience of the practitioner and that throughout this book the term physical therapy is used to describe the treatment, not necessarily the practitioner.

GALLOWAY'S INJURY PREVENTION TOOLS

THE GALLOWAY RUN–WALK–RUN METHOD

"Walk breaks let you control the amount of fatigue and aggravation on your weak links."

Walk breaks have allowed runners with serious injuries to continue running for decades. Those who have had repeat injuries have run injury free when adjusting the run-walk-run ratios. Overall, I've not found any training component that has reduced injury rate while speeding recovery better than this method.

Walk Before You Get Tired

Most of us, even when injured, can walk for several miles before fatigue sets in because walking is an activity that we are bioengineered to do for hours. Running is harder because you must lift your body off the ground and then absorb the shock of the landing, over and over. It's a well-known scientific fact that continuous use of the running muscles, tendons, and joints leads to increased fatigue and more injuries. But if you walk before your running muscles start to get tired or worn, you allow the muscle to recover instantly, increasing your capacity for exercise while reducing the chance that your weak links will get aggravated.

The method part involves having a strategy. By using a ratio that has enough walking for that day, you can keep erasing the fatigue and stress. Those who are experiencing aches and pains should never get locked into any ratio. When stress builds up, walk more.

"The run-walk method is very simple: You run for a short segment, then take a walk break, and keep repeating this pattern."

Walk breaks

- give you control over the way you feel at the end;
- allow older runners and heavier runners to cover any distance they wish and recover fast;
- erase fatigue;
- push back your fatigue wall;
- allow for endorphins to collect during each walk break so that you feel good;
- break up the distance into manageable units ("two more minutes");
- speed recovery;
- reduce the chance of aches, pains, and injury;
- allow you to feel good afterward while performing daily activities you need to do after the run; and
- give you all of the endurance of the distance of each session without the pain.

A Short and Gentle Walking Stride

It's better to walk slowly with a short stride. There has been some irritation of the shins when runners or walkers maintain a stride that is too long. Relax and enjoy the walk.

How to Keep Track of the Walk Breaks

Smartwatches have great apps that can time your intervals. Check my Jeff Galloway Run Walk Run app, available through the app store.

Run-Walk-Run Ratios

After having coached over 500,000 runners, I've come up with the following suggested ratios.

Pace per mile (in minutes)	Run amount	Walk amount
7:00	4 minutes	20 seconds
7:30	4 minutes	25 seconds
8:00	4 minutes	30 seconds
8:30	4 minutes	45 seconds
9:00	4 minutes	60 seconds
9:30	3 minutes	45 seconds
10:00–11:30	3 minutes	60 seconds
11:30–13:00	2 minutes 30 seconds	60 seconds
13:00–14:00	1 minutes	1 minute (or run 30 seconds and walk 30 seconds)
14:00–15:00	30 seconds	30 seconds
15:00–16:00	30 seconds	60 seconds
16:00–17:00	20 seconds	40 seconds
17:00–18:00	15 seconds	45 seconds

In general, I've found that older and heavier runners benefit more from shorter running segments with more frequent walk breaks even when the walks are shorter.

NOTE: While experiencing an injury or coming back after a layoff, it is always better to walk even more than the table would suggest. Many of my athletes will start with a 10-second jog/50-second walk for the first week or two before moving to 15/45, 20/40, and so on. This allows the feet, legs, tendons, and muscles to adapt to the running motion in a gentle way.

USING THE RIGHT PACE AND RUN–WALK–RUN RATIO TO REDUCE INJURY RISK

The training mistake that most commonly leads to injury is running too fast during a race, a long training run, or during a series of speed workouts. By using the magic mile (MM) as a reality check on pacing, you can set a pace and a run-walk-run-ratio for long runs that significantly reduces stress on your weak links and almost eliminates the chance of injury from this key area.

The MM can also tell you what is a realistic goal for the season. Many of the injuries that come from speed training are due to runners choosing a goal that is too ambitious, requiring a speedwork pace that is beyond current capabilities.

The regular insertion of MMs into your training schedule takes the guesswork out of goal setting. Most of my training books have detailed instruction on how to find your MM. My book *The Run Walk Run Method®, Third Edition*, is a great resource.

The Magic Mile

This one-mile time trial (TT) has become my favorite evaluation tool because it is easy to do and has been very accurate. Here's how it works.

1. Go to a track, or other accurately measured course.

2. Warm up by walking for 5 minutes, then running 1 minute and walking 1 minute, then jogging an easy 800 meters (half mile or two laps around a track).

3. Do 4 x 50–yard accelerations that pick up your pace, but not as fast as a sprint.

4. Walk for approximately 2 minutes. Then run the MM, timing yourself for 4 laps. Start your watch at the beginning and keep it running until the end of the fourth lap.

5. On your first MM, don't run all-out from the start—ease into your pace after the first half (2 laps).

6. Cool down by reversing the warm-up.

7. A school track is the best venue. Don't use a treadmill because they tend to be notoriously uncalibrated, and often tell you that you ran farther or faster than you really did.

8. For each successive MM, adjust pace in order to run a faster time than you did on the previous one. By the third or fourth MM, most runners tend to be running very close to their current fastest pace for four laps.

9. Use the following formula to see what time is predicted in the goal races.

10. Add 2 to 3 minutes per mile to the predicted pace for your long runs (3 minutes is better).

Prediction Formulas

To predict your current per mile potential in an all-out effort for longer distances, use the following formulas. To run the resulting time, the following is assumed:

- You have done the training necessary for the goal according to the training programs in The Run Walk Run Method®, Galloway's 5K/10K Running, Galloway's Half Marathon Training, or Running: Getting Started.

- You are not injured.

- You run with an even-paced effort.

- The weather on goal race day is perfect, including 60 °F (14 °C) or cooler.

- You are not running in a crowded race.

- Since this is an ideal prediction, reality is that race times are about 10 to 20 seconds/mile slower than this.

5K: Take your one-mile time and add 33 seconds.

10K: Take your one-mile time and multiply by 1.15.

Half marathon: Take your one-mile time and multiply by 1.2.

Marathon: Take your one-mile time and multiply by 1.3.

Long run pace: 2-3 minutes per mile slower than predicted marathon pace.

EXAMPLE:

Mile time: 10:00

For 5K time, add 33 seconds: 10:33 is predicted mile pace for a 5K.

For 10K time, multiply 10 x 1.15 = 11:30 per mile.

For half marathon time, multiply 10 x 1.2 = 12:00 per mile.

For marathon time, multiply 10 x 1.3 = 13:00 per mile.

Long run pace should be 15-16 min/ per mile.

The "Leap of Faith" Goal Prediction

It is okay to choose a time for your goal race (four to six months in the future) which is faster than is predicted by your pretest. Since you are starting three to six months ahead of the goal race, you can expect to improve by doing the speed training, the long runs, and the drills. For prediction purposes, as you take this "leap" to a goal, I suggest no more than a 5% improvement. First-timers in any race should run to finish. Shoot for a time goal in the second or third race.

- Run the Magic Mile.
- Use the previous formulas to predict what you could run now if you were trained for the goal distance.
- Choose the amount of improvement during program (1-5%).
- Subtract this from # 2—this is your goal time.

Note: In a marathon, the most improvement that I usually see is 30 seconds a mile over a six-month training program (13 minutes). Most time-goal athletes improve 10 minutes or less. Those who attempt a goal that exceeds the prediction formulas put themselves at risk for injury due to the speed required during speedwork.

Final Reality Check

Take your best time during the season and use the prediction formula noted for your goal race. If the resulting prediction is slower than the goal you've been training for, adjust your race goal accordingly. It is strongly recommended that you run the first one-third of your goal race 15 to 20 seconds a mile slower than the pace predicted by the test average.

Slow Down as Temperature Increases

When you exercise strenuously in even moderate heat (above 60 °F/14 °C), you raise your core body temperature. Most beginning runners will see the internal temperature rise above 55 °F/12 °C. This triggers a release of blood into the capillaries of your skin to help cool you down. The reduced oxygen available reduces blood flow to your muscles.

Hot weather slowdown for long runs

As the temperature rises above 55 °F (12 °C), your body starts to incur heat stress, but most runners aren't significantly slowed until 60 °F. If you make the adjustments early, you won't have to suffer later and slow down a lot more at that time. The baseline for this table is 60 °F or 14 °C.

Between 60 and 64 °F	30 seconds/mile slower than you would run at 60 °F
Between 14 and 16.5 °C	20 seconds/kilometer slower than you would run at 14 °C
Between 65 and 69 °F	1 minute/mile slower than you would run at 60 °F
Between 17 and 19.5 °C	40 seconds/kilometer slower than you would run at 14 °C
Between 70 and 74 °F	2 minutes/mile slower than you would run at 60 °F
Between 22.5 and 25 °C	1:20/kilometer slower than you would run at 14 °C
Between 75 and 79 °F	2 minutes/mile slower than you would run at 60 °F
Between 22.5 and 25 °C	1:20/kilometer slower than you would run at 14 °C
Above 80 °F and above 25 °C	Be careful and take extra precautions to avoid heat disease. Or exercise indoors.

CHOOSING THE BEST SHOE FOR YOU

The best advice I can give you is to get the best advice. If you have a good technical running store in your area, go there. The advice you can receive from experienced shoe fitters will be priceless. Here are some other helpful tips.

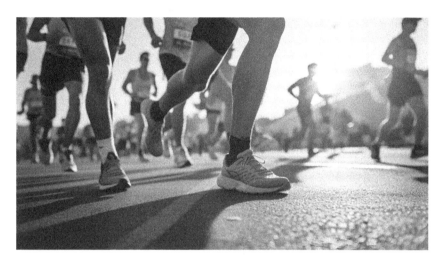

Look at the wear pattern on your most worn pair of walking or running shoes. Use the following tips to help you choose about three pairs of shoes from one of the categories, and compare them:

Floppy feet have spots of wear, including some wear on the inside of the forefoot.

If you have spots of wear and have some foot or knee pain, select a shoe that has minimal cushion or is designed for motion control.

Overpronated foot.

This wear pattern shows significant wear on the inside of the forefoot. If there is knee or hip pain, look for a shoe that has "structure" or motion-control capabilities. If you don't have pain, look at a neutral shoe that does not have a lot of cushion in the forefoot.

Rigid.

If you have a wear pattern on the outside (with some in the middle) of the forefoot of the shoe, and no wear on the inside, you probably have a rigid foot and can choose a neutral shoe that has adequate cushion and flexibility for you, as you run and walk in them.

Go by fit and not the size noted on the box of the shoe.

Most runners wear a running shoe that is about two sizes larger than their street shoe. For example, I wear a size 10 street shoe but run in a size 12 running model. Be open to getting the best fit regardless of what size you see on the running shoe box.

Extra room for your toes.

Your foot tends to swell during the day, so it's best to fit your shoes after noontime. Be sure to stand up in the shoe during the fitting process to measure how much extra room you have in the toe region of the shoe. Pay attention to the longest of your feet, and leave at least half an inch.

Unsure and have no aches or pains.

Choose shoes that are neutral or have a mid-range of cushion and support.

1. Set aside at least 30 minutes to choose your next shoe, as you compare the three candidates you have chosen.

2. Run and walk on a pavement surface to compare the shoes. If you have a floppy foot, make sure that you get the support you need.

3. You want a shoe that feels natural on your foot—no pressure or aggravation—while allowing the foot to go through the range of motion needed for running. Runners that need motion control will feel more firm support from the shoe.

4. Again, take as much time as you need before deciding. If the store doesn't let you run in the shoe, go to another store.

Width Issues

- Running shoes tend to be a bit wider than street shoes.

- Usually, if your foot is a bit narrower, the lacing can "snug up" the difference.

- The shoe shouldn't be laced too tightly around your foot because the foot swells while running and walking. On hot days, the average runner will move up one-half shoe size.

- In general, running shoes are designed to handle a certain amount of "looseness." But if you are getting blisters when wearing a loose shoe, tighten the laces.

- Some shoe companies have selected shoes in widths.

- The shoe is too narrow if you are rolling off the edge of the shoe as you push off on either side.

Shoes for Women

Women's shoes tend to be slightly narrower than those for men, and the heel is usually a bit smaller. The quality of the major running shoe brands is equal (men's models vs women's models). About 25% of women runners have feet that can fit better into men's shoes. Usually the confusion comes when women wear large sizes. The better running stores can help you make a choice in this area.

Breaking in a New Shoe

- Wear the new shoe around the house for an hour or more each day for a week. If you stay on carpet, and the shoe doesn't fit correctly, you can exchange it at the store. But if you have put some wear on the shoe or get them dirty, few stores will take it back.

- In most cases you will find that the shoe feels comfortable enough to run in it immediately. It is best to continue walking in the shoe, gradually allowing the foot to accommodate to the arch, the heel, the ankle pads, and to make other adjustments. If you run in the shoe too soon, blisters are often the result.

- If there are no rubbing issues on the foot when walking, you could walk in the new shoe for a gradually increasing amount for two to four days.

- On the first run, just run about half a mile in the shoe. Put on your old shoes and continue the run.

- On each successive run, increase the distance run in the new shoe for three to four runs. At this point, you will usually have the new shoe broken in.

How do you know when it's time to get a new shoe?

1. When you have been using a shoe for three to four weeks successfully, buy another pair of exactly the same model, make, and size. Shoe companies often make significant changes or discontinue shoe models (even successful ones) every six to eight months.

2. Walk around the house in the new shoe for a few days.

3. After the shoe feels broken in, run the first half mile of one of your weekly runs (shoe break-in day) in the new shoe, then put on the shoe that is already broken in.

4. On this weekly shoe comparison, gradually run a little more in the new shoe.

5. Several weeks later you will notice that the new shoe offers more bounce than the old one.

6. When the old shoe doesn't offer the support you need, shift to the new pair.

7. Start breaking in a third pair.

Credits

Cover and interior design: Anja Elsen

Layout: Anja Elsen

Cover photo: © AdobeStock

Interior photos: © AdobeStock, unless otherwise noted

Managing editor: Elizabeth Evans